QBASE ANAESTHESIA: 2

MCQs FOR THE FINAL FRCA

QBASE ANAESTHESIA: 2
MCQs FOR THE FINAL FRCA

Edited by

Edward Hammond MA BM BCh MRCP FRCA
Shackleton Department of Anaesthetics
Southampton University Hospital NHS Trust

Andrew McIndoe MB ChB FRCA
Sir Humphry Davy Department of Anaesthesia
Bristol Royal Infirmary

Contributors
Mark Blunt
John Isaac
Ravi Gill
Mike Herbertson
Sundeep Karadia
Elfyn Thomas
Gareth Wrathall

GMM

© 1997
Greenwich Medical Media Ltd.
219 The Linen Hall
162-168 Regent Street
London
W1R 5TB

ISBN 1 900151 324

First Published 1997

A catalogue record for this book is available from the British Library

Distributed worldwide by
Oxford University Press

Produced and Designed by
Derek Virtue, DataNet

Printed in Great Britain

CONTENTS

QBase Anaesthesia on CD-ROM

FOREWORD

What do we know? We know that organisations responsible for setting standards who are accountable to the general public must be able to assess their trainees formally. One method is by the FRCA examination which provides, from 1996, two (primary and final) opportunities for summative assessment to complete local appraisal and assessment. These examinations may present significant hurdles in the shortened training programme as only four attempts at each are allowed.

We also know that candidates may be unprepared for these hurdles. There is currently little excuse for this predicament and many sources of help and advice are available from College Tutors, viva practice and writing questions under examination conditions. More difficult perhaps is practice at MCQ papers which can be a threatening test of breadth of knowledge.

First the candidate needs to learn and then test his knowledge and *MCQ technique* ideally in a way which provides feedback leading to improved performance. Prospective candidates are fortunate. This book by Dr. Andrew McIndoe and Dr. Edward Hammond supplies 5 well constructed MCQ examinations of 90 questions covering the syllabus required for the Final FRCA examination. Not only that, explanations of the answers are provided with references so the candidates can identify their areas of weakness and whether their guesswork is a benefit or not. The accompanying interactive CD-ROM allows detailed structured analysis of *performance* and *exam technique* targeted to identify gaps in knowledge which should be addressed.

I congratulate the authors. This book complements their earlier publication on the primary examination and both provide a valuable learning experience for trainees. They should be used repeatedly to improve exam technique in answering MCQ papers in order to ensure a good mark in this part of the examination.

Practice makes perfect; we do at least know that practice with feedback will improve outcome.

SHEILA M. WILLATTS
Consultant in Charge ITU,
Bristol Royal Infirmary
Vice President
Royal College of Anaesthetists
June 1997

INTRODUCTION

The Examination

There are four sections to the Final FRCA examination: a 90 question MCQ paper; a three hour SAQ paper; a fifty minute 'Clinical Anaesthesia' Viva and a thirty minute 'Clinical Science' Viva. Each is evaluated using a four point close-marking system. 2+ is awarded for a good pass; 2 for a pass; 1+ a fail; and 1 is a poor fail. In order to pass overall, a candidate must score 2,2,2,1+ or better and must attempt all the short questions. Thus, relative success is required in all parts of the examination.

The MCQ

Three hours are allowed for the multiple choice paper. This equates to approximately two minutes per question. An enormous amount of mystique surrounds the MCQ, partly because the College does not release past examples of questions. So what is the best strategy to ensure success? First and foremost it is a test of breadth of knowledge. Each paper poses 450 individual problems in the form of 90 questions with 5 parts. No other form of examination is able to cover such ground within the time constraints of a three hour sitting. Thus, the primary aim must be to cover the syllabus which is freely available from the College and forms the basis of this book. Arguments against an MCQ examination system are that it fails to differentiate between rote learning and conceptual appreciation. It has been claimed that the MCQ assessment itself generates cohorts of candidates who have learned to perform well in that particular style of examination, failing in its intended role of assessing competence. Whilst it is true that an examination should transparently reflect the abilities of the candidate without prejudicing those not versed with the system of examination, the reality of the situation is that practice of the technique undoubtedly improves performance. On the other hand the College claims to make every effort to validate each portion of the examination by retrospectively streaming each year group and examining the performance of each band on every question. Those questions that have poor discriminating power or a tendency to invert the groupings are withdrawn. Consistency between year groups is maintained by the use of tried and tested moderator questions that allow inter-year comparisons to be made before defining the cut-off point between success and failure within an exam group. Thus, it is hoped that each candidates performance is assessed objectively, independently and without bias. So what does this mean in terms of technique? Firstly there can be no predetermined pass mark, or for that matter a predetermined pass ratio, since each year group is examined against past year groups. This means that a calculated approach based on number of questions answered correctly is fundamentally flawed. One should attempt as many questions as possible to ensure the maximum chance of success. But what of guessing? The College employs a negative marking system which reduces the potential benefits of guessing. Thus if the examination were presented in Ancient Greek, the majority of candidates would score zero overall. But it is not presented in a foreign language and the dilemma of uncertainty is therefore difficult to negotiate successfully. Few candidates are truly aware of the influences exerted by their own personalities on their examination performance. The world is made up from wild gamblers, play safers and every shade of grey in between these two extremes. It is perhaps surprising that few candidates attempt any form of self assessment prior to tackling a negatively marked paper.

The CD-ROM

The unique interactive CD-ROM enclosed with this book allows detailed analyses of exam performance and technique to be achieved at the push of a button. Examinations have been constructed in the College style using material that covers the entire published syllabus. The 500 questions (each with 5 parts) on the CD can be shuffled and reassembled in an infinite number of exam combinations allowing you to concentrate on specific subjects or to create new exams in the College style. Each question is accompanied by explanatory notes and a reference to an accepted and accessible revision source. When you have completed an exam, the paper is marked before your eyes and your performance objectively assessed, with the option to jump straight to the notes accompanying those questions you may have answered badly. Any exam can be saved to your hard disk or you may simply print a report detailing your performance. The intention has been to construct a versatile interactive safety net that can rapidly identify holes in knowledge that require further revision. Try not to concentrate on the overall mark scored, it is the areas of weakness that matter more. Use of the unique confidence option automates the time-honoured process of labelling answers with different coloured pens to assess MCQ examination technique. Some will be surprised by their over confidence, most will be encouraged by their intuitive skills. This is not merely an attempt to beat the system by playing the odds but rather a positive step towards eliminating the negative effects of poor examination technique that the individual candidate may not have been aware of. The preparation for Collegiate examinations is often a difficult juggling act for trainees, all of whom are required to perform a service commitment and many of whom are coming to terms with the domestic demands of a young family. With available revision time at a premium, Q-Base will help you to rapidly identify areas of weakness and ensure that you approach the negatively marked MCQ examination with a personalised technique least likely to result in failure.

QBase Anaesthesia on CD-ROM has been designed to be easy to use. No knowledge of computers is necessary. It will help you maximise your score. The exam analysis in this version has been substantially enhanced to give you a subject based as well as overall analysis. This new CD will automatically update the version of the program released with QBase 1.

Good luck!

Dr E. Hammond
Dr A. McIndoe
July 1997

Exam 1

QUESTION 1

The initial management of a patient with suspected anaphylaxis during anaesthesia includes

A. 50% oxygen
B. 0.5 - 1.0 ml of adrenaline 1:10,000 intramuscularly
C. 0.5 - 1.0 mg of adrenaline intravenously at a rate of 0.5 mg/minute until a response is obtained
D. Chlorpheniramine 10 - 20 mg by slow intravenous injection
E. Hydrocortisone 100 - 300 mg intravenously

QUESTION 2

Atmospheric pressure can be quoted as approximately

A. 76 cmHg
B. 15 lb/in^2
C. 100 Nm
D. 1 bar
E. 7.6 mH$_2$O

QUESTION 3

In deep vein thrombosis

A. Platelets form the greatest bulk of the thrombus
B. Sickle cell anaemia is a cause
C. A positive Homan's sign is diagnostic
D. Pulmonary embolism is commonest with thromboses below the knee
E. Destruction of vein valves is accompanied by oedema

QUESTION 4

The body's intracellular buffers consist primarily of

A. Haemoglobin
B. Proteins
C. Albumin
D. Creatinine
E. Polypeptides

QUESTION 5

For patients receiving anaesthesia at increased altitude

A. Atmospheric pressure decreases linearly with increasing altitude

B. Hyperpnoea enhances oxygen uptake in the lungs and its offloading in the tissues

C. At 10,000 feet 50% nitrous oxide will be less analgesic than at sea level

D. For the same minute ventilation, work of breathing will be reduced compared to sea-level

E. Halothane vapourisers will have to be manually adjusted to compensate for altered atmospheric pressure

QUESTION 6

The following drugs should be administered at reduced dosages to patients with impaired renal function

A. Azaproprazone

B. Enalapril

C. Atenolol

D. Frusemide

E. Cefuroxime

QUESTION 7

Cardioversion is indicated in

A. Ventricular tachycardia

B. Asystole

C. Atrial flutter

D. Digoxin toxicity

E. Bundle branch block

QUESTION 8

A systolic murmur is classically present in

A. Mitral stenosis

B. Tricuspid stenosis

C. Atrial septal defect

D. Mitral regurgitation

E. Pulmonary hypertension

QUESTION 9

Hyperglycaemia may result from the administration of

A. Adrenaline

B. Thyroid stimulating hormone

C. Beta blockers

D. Thiazide diuretics

E. Glucagon

QUESTION 10

Concerning diathermy

A. Direct current with a frequency 1 MHz is used
B. Employs a low current density at the site of intended tissue damage
C. Bipolar diathermy requires more power than unipolar diathermy
D. Is contraindicated if the patient has a pacemaker
E. May cause burns at the site of plate application

QUESTION 11

In patients who require carotid endarterectomy

A. Cerebral autoregulation is often shifted to the right
B. Cerebral blood flow varies directly with arterial oxygen content
C. Cerebral blood flow varies in an exponential manner with $PaCO_2$
D. Cerebral blood flow is affected by blood viscosity and age
E. Hypoxia increases cerebral blood flow

QUESTION 12

Auditory Evoked Potentials (AEPs)

A. Brainstem AEPs are used to monitor depth of anaesthesia
B. Because the measurement lasts 80-100 msec, up to ten independent measurements can be made each second
C. Changes in AEPs are mostly independent of the anaesthetic agent in use
D. AEPs of latency 15-80 msec are of value for monitoring Posterior Fossa surgery
E. AEPs require a silent operating theatre for their successful application

QUESTION 13

Considering a frequent social user of cocaine for general anaesthesia

A. Myocardial ischaemia occurs due to contaminant induced coronary artery disease
B. Chronic use of the drug lowers the seizure threshold
C. Chronic pulmonary problems are unlikely
D. A dose of Brompton cocktail could be an ideal pre-medicant
E. Hypertension and tachycardia preoperatively should not be treated

QUESTION 14

Using the 'Tec 6' vapouriser for desflurane

A. The sump is heated to provide a vapour pressure of 10% above atmospheric pressure
B. The vapour circuit gas flow is not determined by the fresh gas flow
C. Compensation for changes in atmospheric pressure are by manual adjustment
D. The working pressure of the vapouriser increases linearly with increased fresh gas flow
E. Is not possible in event of a power failure

QUESTION 15

In the treatment of epilepsy

A. Thiopentone is the first line drug in status epilepticus

B. Phenytoin may be administered intravenously at a rate not exceeding 100 mg/min in an adult

C. Concurrent administration of phenytoin may increase the plasma concentration of phenobarbitone

D. Lamotrigine therapy should be started with a loading dose

E. Carbamazepine may cause hypernatraemia

QUESTION 16

Concerning pulmonary embolism (PE) and its management

A. About 60 % are thought to arise in the deep veins of the lower extremities and pelvis

B. Pulmonary angiography is the diagnostic gold standard

C. Cyanosis is common

D. An associated bradycardia is a good prognostic sign

E. Frusemide should be given to aid oxygenation

QUESTION 17

Renal sodium wasting may result from

A. Bilateral renal vascular disease

B. Nephrotic syndrome

C. Diabetic nephropathy

D. Addison's disease

E. Lithium therapy

QUESTION 18

Cushings Disease is associated with

A. Obesity

B. Hypertension

C. Distal muscle wasting

D. Menorrhagia

E. Depression

QUESTION 19

Considering the use of peripheral nerve stimulators

- **A.** Force of contraction continues to rise above the maximal stimulation threshold
- **B.** Fade is a characteristic of depolarizing blockade
- **C.** Double burst stimulation involves the use of two consecutive trains of four stimuli
- **D.** Double burst stimuli should be separated by 0.75 seconds
- **E.** A train of four stimuli are normally delivered at 0.5Hz

QUESTION 20

The following have autosomal dominant inheritance

- **A.** Hereditary spherocytosis
- **B.** Motor neurone disease
- **C.** Duchenne muscular dystrophy
- **D.** Myasthenia gravis
- **E.** Acute intermittent porphyria

QUESTION 21

Concerning the diagnosis of pneumonia

- **A.** H. influenzae is the commonest community acquired pathogen
- **B.** Q fever is caught from farm animals
- **C.** Endotracheal aspirates correlate poorly with LRTI
- **D.** Recent influenza infection indicates the need for particular cover against Legionella pneumophilia
- **E.** Ventilator acquired Pseudomonas aeruginosa infection has a high mortality

QUESTION 22

In the management of cerebral oedema

- **A.** Mannitol is more effective than frusemide
- **B.** Mannitol works more quickly than hyperventilation
- **C.** Fluid restriction requires several days to have an effect
- **D.** Steroids are of benefit in patients with tumours
- **E.** Frusemide causes greater electrolyte abnomalities than mannitol

QUESTION 23

Concerning the effects of a 'massive' transfusion

- **A.** The commonest abnormality is an elevated INR
- **B.** The plasma level of factor V falls in proportion to the volume transfused
- **C.** Following a single blood volume replacement procoagulant levels are below 20% of their normal levels
- **D.** Diffuse microvascular bleeding is related to low procoagulant levels
- **E.** A fibrinogen level of 100 mg/dl is an indication for FFP in a bleeding patient

QUESTION 24

Considering lactate metabolism

A. Increase in plasma lactate will be matched by an equal mmolar decrease in plasma bicarbonate

B. Fitness training does not affect the rate of rise in plasma lactate

C. Glucose metabolism to lactate releases ATP at the same rate as oxidation within the mitochondria

D. After exercise lactate is largely reconverted into glucose

E. Lactate filtered in the kidney is actively reabsorbed

QUESTION 25

In acute pancreatitis

A. Contrast enhanced CT scans are of no use in diagnosing pancreatic necrosis

B. Infected pancreatic necrosis should be aspirated percutaneously under ultrasound control

C. Grey Turner's sign describes umbilical ecchymoses

D. The cause is most commonly gallstones or alcohol

E. The APACHE II score should be calculated to predict mortality

QUESTION 26

The following ion compositions are correct

A. 0.9% saline - sodium 131 mmol/l

B. Albumin 4.5% – calcium 2 mmol/l

C. Hartmann's solution - chloride 154 mmol/l

D. Gelofusine - calcium 5.1 mmol/l

E. Dextrose 4% saline 0.18% - sodium 30 mmol/l

QUESTION 27

The following are true concerning humidity and humidification of gases

A. Relative humidity is the ratio of absolute humidity to saturated humidity at a specified temperature

B. Operating theatre humidity should be maintained at no more than 30%

C. Heat and moisture exchangers can achieve 40% humidity

D. A nebuliser works on the poiseuille effect to entrain water across a pressure drop

E. The water trap for a simple bottle humidifier must be as larger as the humidifier bottle

QUESTION 28

Concerning humidification of inspired gases

A. Under normal circumstances, the relative humidity in the upper trachea is 40%

B. Ciliary clearance continues normally until the relative humidity falls below 24%

C. Heat and moisture exchangers (HMEs) are recommended for paediatric use

D. Water reservoirs are particularly at risk of contamination with Pseudomonas species

E. Ultrasonic nebulisers produce optimal humidification

QUESTION 29

The following agents decrease the heart rate

A. Diltiazem
B. Neostigmine
C. Hydralazine
D. Nifedipine
E. Halothane

QUESTION 30

In a patient with a traumatic cervical spinal cord transection

A. Spinal shock has usually resolved within a week of injury
B. Hypertension may be present pre-operatively
C. Hypertension in response to surgical stimulation below the level of the transection is unlikely
D. There is increased sensitivity to ACE inhibitors
E. Positive pressure ventilation is more likely to cause bradycardia

QUESTION 31

When considering weaning from mechanical ventilation

A. In the majority of patients, a PaO_2/FiO_2 ratio of less than 200 is a prerequisite
B. If spontaneous respiratory frequency divided by the Vt (in litres) < 80, a successful wean is unlikely
C. Hypophosphataemia should be corrected to improve respiratory muscle strength
D. The maximum negative pressure generated during inspiration assesses the respiratory muscle strength
E. Auto-PEEP makes failure more likely because it reduces the respiratory drive

QUESTION 32

Serum Na$^+$ 120 mmol/l and K$^+$ 6.4 mmol/l are consistent with

A. Hyperaldosteronism
B. Renal failure
C. Hypopituitarism
D. Adrenocortical insufficiency
E. Cushings disease

QUESTION 33

Concerning the management of drowning

A. Steroids improve outcome if given in the first 48 hours
B. Sodium bicarbonate will improve the acidosis and thus myocardial function
C. ICP monitoring is a clinically useful tool
D. Rapid re-warming may result in circulatory collapse
E. If comatosed on arrival at hospital, adults have a lower mortality than children

QUESTION 34

Concerning the use of a Sengstaken-Blakemore tube to control variceal bleeding

A. Bleeding is generally controlled with an oesophageal balloon
B. The gastric ballon should be inflated with 500 mls of air
C. If endotracheal intubation is required, it needs to be performed after the tube is in position
D. Traction on the tube should be equivalent a 300-500 g mass
E. Chest pains suggest rebleeding and the balloons should be inflated with 50 ml aliquots until this stops

QUESTION 35

The kidneys

A. Receive 25% of the cardiac output
B. Do not allow the glomerular filtration rate to vary
C. In a healthy adult will produce up to 180 litres of glomerular filtrate per day
D. Consume 15ml of oxygen per 100g tissue each minute
E. Oxygen consumption is dependent upon blood flow

QUESTION 36

In the measurement of gas flow

A. The rotameter is a variable pressure, variable orifice device
B. The pneumotacograph is used to measure turbulent flow
C. In a rotameter at low flow rates, flow is a function of density
D. The bobbin of a Heidbrink flowmeter rotates
E. Readings are taken from the bottom of the bobbin in the rotameter

QUESTION 37

In positioning patients during anaesthesia

A. In the spontaneously breathing patient ventilation to the lower lung will be greater
B. Tilted patients with sympathetic dystrophies are at risk of organ hypoperfusion
C. In lithotomy pressure on the medial tibial condyle may damage the saphenous nerve
D. There should be no more than a 90 degree angle between body and arm
E. The sitting position is not a greater risk for venous air embolism than lying flat

QUESTION 38

Peptic ulceration

A. Is commoner in patients with blood group A
B. Is associated with hypoparathyroidism
C. Incidence is increased in smokers
D. Duodenal ulcers occur most commonly in the 2nd part
E. Duodenal ulcer pain is classically relieved by food

QUESTION 39

The Apgar score

A. Was developed by paediatricians as a neonatal outcome tool
B. Should be performed at 1 and 10 minutes after birth
C. Includes an assessment of muscle tone
D. Has a maximum score of 10
E. Scores are from 0-3 for each parameter

QUESTION 40

Ventilatory failure is commonly associated with

A. A decrease in functional residual capacity
B. Increased lung and total thoracic compliance
C. Increased lung water
D. Chest wall abnormalities
E. An adequate arterial oxygen content

QUESTION 41

Pre-eclampsia

A. Is associated with polyhydramnios and multiple pregnancy
B. Complicates 22% of all pregnancies
C. Is a contraindication to extradural anaesthesia if the platelet count is <100000
D. Is a single system disorder associated with hypertension
E. If complicated by cerebral irritation is treated with magnesium sulphate

QUESTION 42

An increase in left ventricular myocardial contractility

A. Can be measured by changes in maximum dp/dt in the left ventricle over a range of blood pressures
B. Will increase cardiac output and so decrease any risk of myocardial ischaemia
C. Is a reflex response to an increase in heart rate
D. Is demonstrated by a decrease in left ventricular end systolic elastance
E. Occurs when left ventricular afterload is acutely lowered

QUESTION 43

Activated coagulation time

A. Is normally 25-49 seconds
B. Requires 2 ml of blood
C. Is 'activated' by kaolin
D. Is linearly prolonged in proportion to the dose of heparin administered
E. Is prolonged by hypothermia

QUESTION 44

Fibreoptic bronchoscopy in a mechanically ventilated patient

A. Will not reduce the expired minute volume if the ventilator is of the volume controlled type

B. Should be performed by a respiratory physician

C. Is not useful for the removal of foreign bodies

D. Has no effect on the level of PEEP delivered

E. Can result in hypoxia that lasts for several hours

QUESTION 45

Coeliac Plexus Block

A. Is a useful method of treating intractable pain accompanying carcinoma of the pancreas

B. Denervates the foregut

C. Is performed bilaterally at L2

D. Is performed anterolateral to the abdominal aorta

E. Is most commonly complicated by postural hypotension

QUESTION 46

Remifentanil

A. Has a similar potency to fentanyl

B. Does not cause muscle rigidity

C. Is predominantly broken down by plasma cholinesterase

D. Has a recovery time more rapid than alfentanil following intravenous infusion

E. Is a pure mu receptor agonist

QUESTION 47

The Myasthenic patient

A. Requires neuromuscular blockade for a thymectomy

B. Is more likely to display symptoms of toxicity following ester local anaesthesia

C. Is prone to tachydysrhythmias peroperatively

D. Is more sensitive to suxamethonium

E. Is more likely to develop Phase II block in response to suxamethonium

QUESTION 48

Concerning the use of hydroxyethyl starch as an intravenous fluid

A. Glomerular filtration is the major route of elimination

B. About 48% of the total dose is deposited in the reticuloendothelial system (RES)

C. Large volumes may alter coagulation by lowering factor X concentrations

D. The incidence of allergic reactions is similar to that of the gelatins

E. Serum amylase concentrations may be elevated up to threefold following its use

QUESTION 49

The trachea

A. Terminates at T6
B. Has a blood supply from the superior thyroid artery
C. Lateral relations in the neck include the recurrent laryngeal nerve
D. Has no muscular fibres in its structures
E. Anteriorly is always crossed by the thyroid ima artery

QUESTION 50

Acute arterial embolisation is characterised by

A. Immobility of the affected limb
B. Pain
C. Loss of pin-prick sensation in the affected limb
D. Pallor
E. Loss of light touch sensation in the affected limb

QUESTION 51

Concerning echocardiography

A. Blood flow velocity within the heart is normally >1 m/s
B. Pressure difference across a valve is calculated from blood velocity
C. M mode is useful for assessing timing of events
D. Colourflow Doppler has replaced two dimensional echocardiography
E. Doppler echocardiography records a change in amplitude of ultrasound reflected from moving red cells

QUESTION 52

When prescribing total parenteral nutrition (TPN) the daily allowances of nutrients per kg in a normal adult are

A. Glucose 3g
B. Calcium 0.7 - 1.0 mmol
C. Magnesium 0.5 - 0.8 mmol
D. Sodium 1 - 2 mmol
E. Water 30 ml

QUESTION 53

The following are associated

A. Hypothyroidism and oligomenorrhoea
B. Bronchial carcinoma and hyponatraemia
C. Marfans syndrome and a high arched palate
D. Aortic stenosis and sudden death
E. Tetany and hyperparathyroidism

QUESTION 54

The following are recognised causes of diarrhoea in the critically ill patient

A. Digoxin therapy
B. Aluminium containing antacids
C. Mesenteric venous thrombosis
D. Clostridium difficile infection
E. Enteral feed

QUESTION 55

Concerning bradycardias and their management

A. In suspected sinus node disease with a normal ECG the initial investigation of choice is a 24 hour tape
B. Lyme disease may cause acute and permanent heart block
C. Mobitz type 2 second degree heart block is characterized by a progressively lengthening P-R interval
D. Third degree heart block following an inferior myocardial infarction requires a temporary pacemaker
E. The optimal pacemaker mode for sinus node disease is VVI

QUESTION 56

When considering anaesthesia in the radiology department

A. The radiation exposure during CT of head is greater than that for a skull X-ray
B. Laryngoscopes are magnetic
C. Myelography in the paediatric patient requires them to be prone
D. Angiography quality can be enhanced by hyperventilation
E. Contrast media injection can cause wheeze

QUESTION 57

For safe cardio-pulmonary bypass the following are required

A. A heparin dose of 30 units/kg
B. An activated clotting time of greater than 400 seconds
C. Myocardial cooling to less than 32°C for myocardial protection
D. Examination of carotid pulses to ensure their presence and equality after the onset of bypass
E. A reverse trendelenberg positon for the patient if arterial air embolus occurs

QUESTION 58

When using agents to reduce blood pressure

A. Trimetaphan crosses the blood brain barrier and may cause confusion
B. Sodium nitroprusside should be avoided in renal failure
C. Nitroglycerine should be protected from the light
D. Cyanide toxicity following sodium nitroprusside infusion can be treated with dimercaprol
E. Hydralazine exerts its effects by promoting nitric oxide production

QUESTION 59

Haemophilia A is associated with

A. Haemarthrosis
B. Prolonged prothrombin time
C. Normal bleeding time
D. Hepatitis B
E. Successful treatment with desmopressin

QUESTION 60

Repeated enteral doses of activated charcoal enhance the elimination of the following drugs

A. Amitriptyline
B. Warfarin
C. Paracetamol
D. Digoxin
E. Quinine

QUESTION 61

Regarding a variable that has a normal distribution

A. The mode, mean and median will be the same
B. The variance will equal the standard deviation
C. Population means have no relationship to sample means
D. The coefficient of variance is a constant
E. A value greater than two standard deviations from the mean is abnormal

QUESTION 62

Neuromuscular monitoring

A. A T4:T1 ratio of 0.75 means that the patient is suitably reversed for extubation
B. Double burst stimulation is of particular value for monitoring deep relaxation
C. Post-tetanic count is most often used for assessing suitability for extubation
D. Normal neuromuscular function will display no fade with a supramaximal 50Hz stimulus for 5 seconds
E. Tetanic stimulation can be reassessed only once a minute

QUESTION 63

In surgical correction for scoliosis

A. The presence of pulmonary hypertension is a contraindication to surgery
B. Harrington rods may be employed
C. Pre-operative right ventricular hypertrophy is a feature
D. One lung anaesthesia may be necessary
E. A high incidence of intra-operative recall occurs if a 'wake-up' test is employed

QUESTION 64

Gastroduodenal stress ulceration

A. Has become less common over the last 20 years

B. Is more common in certain groups of patients

C. Prevention with antacids is associated with an increased rate of nosocomial pneumonia

D. Causing overt bleeding is present in 40-50% of critically ill patients

E. May be prevented by sucralfate due to its antisecretory actions

QUESTION 65

When managing a confused patient in the intensive care unit

A. Vitamin abnormalities are a possible cause

B. The cause may be the blockage of a urinary catheter

C. Psychiatric referral should be made as soon as possible

D. 'ICU' psychosis can be diagnosed if there is an underlying psychiatric illness

E. The possibility of previous alcohol abuse is unimportant acutely

QUESTION 66

A diagnosis of acute appendicitis in a patient with right iliac fossa pain is unlikely if

A. There is a pyrexia of 40 degrees celsius

B. Pyuria > 1000 WC/mm^3

C. Rovsing's sign is positive

D. The patient is hungry

E. There has previously been central colicky abdominal pain

QUESTION 67

Pseudo-obstruction

A. Is rare in the elderly

B. Is associated with uraemia

C. Should be investigated with barium enema

D. Cannot be treated by colonoscopy

E. Requires diagnostic laparotomy

QUESTION 68

The patient with a proven subarachnoid haemorrhage (SAH)

A. Must have arterial hypertension controlled immediately and aggressively

B. Has a 90% short term mortality if surgery is not undertaken

C. Should have repeat CT scanning if their neurological status gradually deteriorates

D. Will have xanthochromia of the CSF if lumbar puncture is performed within 4 hours of the event

E. Is most prone to vasospasm in the first 5 days

QUESTION 69

Sinus bradycardia occurs with the following

A. Anal dilatation
B. Ophthalmic surgery
C. Skin incision
D. Cervical dilatation
E. Bladder retraction

QUESTION 70

The following are normal values obtained using a flow directed pulmonary artery catheter

A. Cardiac index (CI) 4.5 - 6 L/min/m²
B. Systemic vascular resistance (SVR) 1500 - 2500 dynes s cm⁻⁵
C. Stroke volume (SV) 60 - 120 ml/beat
D. Oxygen delivery (DO₂I) 300 -500 ml/min/m²
E. Left ventricular stroke work (LVSW) 50 - 120 gm/beat

QUESTION 71

In the event of thoracic trauma

A. Thoracotomy is indicated if 1500mls of blood is evacuated from a chest drain inserted for haemothorax
B. Rib fractures, if present, are most likely to involve the first to third ribs
C. Subcutaneous emphysema is found in fracture of the larynx
D. Diaphragmatic rupture is more easily diagnosed on the right
E. Computed tomography is the investigation of choice in suspected aortic injury

QUESTION 72

The following are true of colloids

A. Hetastarch provides longer plasma volume expansion than pentastarch
B. Dextran 70 can have an effect on coagulation due to an anti-thrombin effect on platelets
C. Succinylated gelatins produce less allergic responses than urea-linked versions
D. Haptens are used to decrease the incidence of allergic reactions to starches
E. Physically colloids differ from crystalloid fluids only in the size of molecules

QUESTION 73

Regarding the blood supply to the heart

A. The right coronary artery arises from the posterior aortic sinus
B. The sinoatrial node is usually supplied by the left coronary artery
C. The anterior descending artery is a branch of the left coronary artery
D. In most hearts the atrioventricular node is supplied by the left coronary artery
E. Electrocardiographic ischaemic changes in leads II, III and aVf represent occlusion in the right coronary artery

QUESTION 74

Considering the circulation of blood to the brain

A. Normally the intracranial blood volume is 200 ml in an adult
B. The normal cerebral blood flow is 100 ml/100gm/min
C. The effect of CO_2 on cerebral blood flow is via changes in perivascular pH
D. Cerebral vasodilatation in response to hypoxia is mediated via nitric oxide
E. Cerebral ischaemia becomes clinically apparent when MAP falls below the patients autoregulatory limit

QUESTION 75

In a normal PA chest radiograph

A. The right diaphragm is 2.5 cm lower than the left
B. The cardiac shadow is less than half the thoracic diameter
C. The horizontal fissure lies at the level of T5 posteriorly and the 4th rib anteriorly
D. Radiographic density is independent of rotation
E. The right hilum lies above the left hilum

QUESTION 76

Concerning the pleura

A. Both right and left cross the midaxillary line at the level of the eighth costal cartilage
B. Diaphragmatic pleura is supplied only by the phrenic nerve
C. The lung has the same surface markings as the cervical pleura
D. It is unguarded by ribs at the right xiphisternal angle
E. Lies 2 intercostal spaces below the lower borders of the lungs

QUESTION 77

Concerning spirometric tests

A. Asthma reduces the FEV_1 to a similar extent to the FVC
B. The PEFR provides similar information to the FEV_1
C. The maximum breathing capacity is tested over 30 seconds
D. Pulmonary fibrosis causes the FEV_1 / FVC ratio to be greater than 0.7
E. Normally the FEV_1 is over 75% of the FVC

QUESTION 78

For non invasive measurement of blood pressure

A. The use of an overlapped long cuff causes errors in readings
B. There is overestimation at lower pressures compared with direct measurement
C. The oscillotonometer gives an accurate measurement of diastolic pressure
D. Oscillometric instruments remain accurate in the presence of atrial fibrillation
E. Continuous non invasive blood pressure measurements rely on changes in the blood volume in a finger

QUESTION 79

The following are correct

- **A.** The sternal angle is at the level of the second costal cartilage
- **B.** The highest point of the iliac crest lies at the level of the second lumbar vertebra
- **C.** The spinal anterior longitudinal ligament stretches from the atlas to the fifth piece of the sacrum
- **D.** The oesophagus passes through the diaphragm at the level of the eighth thoracic vertebra
- **E.** The thyroid cartilage lies opposite the sixth cervical vertebra

QUESTION 80

A neonate born at 30 weeks and now 15 weeks old is to have an inguinal hernia repaired

- **A.** Pre-operative milk starvation needs to be no longer than for term neonates
- **B.** The risk of post operative apnoea remains high until a post-conceptual age of 70 weeks
- **C.** The spinal cord ends at a lower level than in adults
- **D.** A sensory level of block up to T10 from a spinal anaesthetic is needed
- **E.** Spinal anaesthesia does not decrease the risk of post-operative apnoea

QUESTION 81

In the function of the autonomic nervous system

- **A.** Preganglionic neurones can be cholinergic or adrenergic
- **B.** Parasympathetic nervous system stimulation produces coronary vasodilatation
- **C.** The stellate ganglia aid myocardial contractility
- **D.** Alpha-2 stimulation modifies intracellular cGMP levels
- **E.** Circulating catecholamines have a t1/2 of 5 minutes

QUESTION 82

Transcutaneous Electrical Nerve Stimulation (TENS)

- **A.** The electrical stimuli act directly on C fibres
- **B.** The impulses should be 0–50 μA in strength
- **C.** The stimulation should not be strong enough for the patient to experience paraesthesia
- **D.** Can be used to treat angina
- **E.** Development of tolerance to the analgesic effect is a common problem

QUESTION 83

Antibacterial prophylaxis

- **A.** For a patient with an ASD undergoing TURP may include a combination of amoxycillin and vancomycin
- **B.** In those having had endocarditis may consist purely of amoxycillin
- **C.** To close contacts of a case of meningococcal meningitis will include phenoxymethylpenicillin
- **D.** Is not required in a patient with mitral stenosis undergoing a Caesarean Section
- **E.** Is unnecessary in a child following splenectomy if they have received HIB vaccine

QUESTION 84

Selective decontamination of the digestive tract (SDD) includes

A. Cefuroxime intravenously for 4 days

B. Amphotericin intravenously for 10 days

C. Tobramycin 80 mg enterally 6 hourly

D. Oral paste containing 2 % amphotericin, colomycin and tobramycin applied 6 hourly

E. Metronidazole 500 mg intravenously for 4 days

QUESTION 85

Pseudomembranous colitis

A. Usually presents 5-10 days after antibiotic therapy

B. Is caused by Clostridium difficile

C. Treatment with vancomycin requires a trough plasma level of 5-10 mg/l

D. Is often recurrent

E. Presents with bloody diarrhoea

QUESTION 86

Concerning bronchial carcinoma

A. Adenocarcinomas are proportionally more common in smokers

B. Can be associated with enophthalmos

C. Tumours of up to 0.5cm can reliably be recognised on chest x-ray

D. Daily treatment with prednisolone is used to reduce oedema formation around the tumour

E. Clubbing is present in 30% of all cases

QUESTION 87

Regarding urological surgery

A. Hypotonic glycine solution is used for irrigation as it will not conduct electricity

B. The irrigation fluid can be safely placed up to 1m above the patient

C. TURP syndrome develops when blood glycine levels reach 60 mmol/l

D. TURP syndrome is more common when warm irrigation fluid is used

E. Transient blindness is a presenting feature of TURP syndrome

QUESTION 88

A poor prognosis following pneumonectomy is predicted by

A. A maximum breathing capcity of <50% predicted

B. An FEV1 of <70% predicted

C. Undergoing a right pneumonectomy as compared to a left pnemonectomy

D. Being older than 60 years of age

E. A $PaCO_2$ of >50 mmHg

QUESTION 89

The following will cause a rise in the SvO$_2$ measured by a fibreoptic PA catheter

A. Acute haemorrhage
B. Starting an adrenaline infusion
C. Wedging of the catheter
D. Mitral value rupture
E. An increase in arterial saturation

QUESTION 90

Colonic carcinoma

A. Is often a squamous carcinoma
B. Duke's B tumour involve the regional lymph nodes
C. Whole blood transfusion should be avoided
D. Is inoperable in 30% of patients
E. Usually presents with obstruction

Exam 1: Answers

ANSWER 1

A. FALSE   B. FALSE   C. FALSE   D. FALSE   E. FALSE

Anaphylactic reactions are rare during anaesthesia. It is estimated that there may be 175 - 1000 reactions in the UK each year. The clinical features of anaphylaxis are cardiovascular collapse, bronchospasm, angio-oedema, generalised oedema and cutaneous signs such as rash, erythema and urticaria. The response to treatment may depend on the severity of the reaction, however even severe anaphylaxis responds promptly to appropriate treatment in most patients. Initial therapy includes:

- Stop administration of suspected drug(s)
- Give 100% oxygen and maintain the airway
- Lay patient flat and elevate the legs
- Give adrenaline: IM - 0.5 - 1.0 mg (0.5 - 1 ml of 1:1,000) repeated every 10 minutes

IV - 50 - 100 mcg (0.5 - 1 ml of 1:10,000) over 1 minute with titration of further doses. In a patient with cardiovascular collapse 0.5 - 1.0 mg may be required intravenously in divided doses by titration at a rate of 0.1 mg/minute until an adequate response is obtained.

- Start IV volume expansion

Secondary therapy includes:

- Antihistamines
- Corticosteroids
- Catecholamine infusions
- Bicarbonate
- Bronchodilators

Ref: Association of Anaesthetists. Suspected Anaphylactic Reactions Associated with Anaesthesia. Revised edition 1995.

ANSWER 2

A. TRUE   B. TRUE   C. FALSE   D. TRUE   E. FALSE

Pressure = Force / Area = N / m^2

1 atmosphere = 1 bar = 760 mmHg = 76 cmHg

Hg has a relative density = 13.6 x H_2O, therefore 760 mmHg = 10.3 mH_2O

Ref: Junior Pears Encyclopaedia!!

ANSWER 3

A. FALSE   B. TRUE   C. FALSE   D. FALSE   E. TRUE

The thrombus of a deep vein thrombosis (DVT) consists mainly of red cells and fibrin (red thrombus). Sickling in sickle cell crises leads to an increased blood viscosity which is associated with both arterial and venous thrombosis. Homan's sign is pain in the calf on dorsiflexion of the foot, and though present in DVT it also occurs with other lesions of the calf. Pulmonary embolism is most common with DVT from an iliofemoral thrombosis and is rare with those below the knee. In DVT, deep vein valve destruction leads to a painful swollen limb, oedema and venous eczema.

Ref: Kumar & Clark. Clinical Medicine. Balliere Tindall. Ch 6, 11

ANSWER 4

A. FALSE   B. TRUE   C. FALSE   D. FALSE   E. TRUE

In a metabolic acidosis with a decreased blood bicarbonate the biochemical findings result from the addition of an acid load to the extracellular compartment and this load may be endogenous or exogenous. The body's response to an acid load includes the titration of this load by various fixed intracellular and extracellular buffers. The intracellular buffers consist primarily of proteins and polypeptides while the extracellular buffers include haemoglobin, bicarbonate, albumin and creatinine.

Ref: Current Anaesthesia and Critical Care 1996; Vol 7, No 4:pg 182-186. Current concepts in acid-base balance: use of bicarbonate in patients with metabolic acidosis.

ANSWER 5

A. FALSE   B. FALSE   C. TRUE   D. TRUE   E. FALSE

There is a non linear relationship between falling atmospheric pressure with rising altitude. Hyperpnoea due to hypoxia will lead to hypocarbia. This results in a left shift of the haemoglobin-oxygen dissociation curve; although this improves the uptake of oxygen by blood in the lungs it makes its offloading in the tissues less efficient. However the overall effect on oxygen transport is beneficial. The analgesic effects of nitrous oxide depend on its absolute partial pressure which will be less for the same % when at increased altitude. The reduced gas density at higher altitude reduces breathing resistance and therefore the work of breathing. Halothane vapourisers compensate for a change in atmospheric pressure and still produce the same partial pressure of halothane in the outflow

Ref: Miller. Anesthesia. Churchill Livingstone. Chapter 71.

ANSWER 6

A. TRUE   B. TRUE   C. TRUE   D. FALSE   E. TRUE

ARF due to NSAIDs and ACE inhibitors is generally haemodynamically mediated. They tend to cause ARF in patients with a low renal blood flow in whom maintenance of an adequate GFR is dependent upon low afferent and high efferent arteriolar tone. NSAIDs inhibit cyclo-oxygenase and so reduce the synthesis of locally produced prostaglandins which dilate the afferent arterioles, while ACE inhibitors decrease the production of angiotensin-2 which constricts the efferent arterioles. Beta blockers need to be given in reduced doses due to their effect on renal blood flow and some, like atenolol, nadolol, pindolol and sotalol are excreted unchanged from the kidney. Most cephalosporins need to be given in reduced dosage in renal impairment. Loop diuretics are used in the treatment and prevention of ARF and have the theoretical advantage of reducing oxygen consumption in the ascending loop of Henle by inhibiting active sodium reabsorption. However they potentiate the nephrotoxicity of many other drugs and if used relatively large doses are required.

Ref: British Journal of Hospital Medicine. 1996, Vol55, No4, pg 162-175. Aspects of renal failure.

ANSWER   7

A. TRUE   B. FALSE   C. TRUE   D. FALSE   E. FALSE

The major difference between cardioversion and defibrillation is that the former is synchronised so that the shock occurs during the downstroke of the QRS complex. In asystole, cardioversion is not indicated unless ventricular fibrillation cannot be excluded. Atrial flutter and fibrillation (of onset less than 1 year) are indications for cardioversion. Digoxin toxicity may lead to ventricular arrythmyias or asystole following cardioversion. Therapeutic digoxin levels do not increase the risks of this but it is conventional to omit digoxin several days prior to planned cardioversion.

Ref: Kumar & Clark. Clinical Medicine. Balliere Tindall. Chapter 11

ANSWER   8

A. FALSE   B. FALSE   C. TRUE   D. TRUE   E. TRUE

In mitral stenosis there is a mid diastolic mumur heard best at the apex. The diastolic mumur in tricuspid stenosis is heard best along the lower sternal edge. In pulmonary hypertension and atrial septal defect the systolic mumur is heard best in the pulmonary area wheras in mitral regurgitation it is at the apex.

Ref: Burton. Aids to Undergraduate Medicine. 3rd edition. Churchill Livingstone.

ANSWER   9

A. TRUE   B. TRUE   C. FALSE   D. TRUE   E. TRUE

Adrenaline increases glucagon and stimulates gluconeogenesis. Patients on beta blockers are at risk of hypoglycaemia under general anaesthesia, whilst thiazide diuretics commonly precipitate NIDDM.

Ref: Scurr, Feldman and Soni. Scientific Foundations 4th ed.pp 371

ANSWER   10

A. FALSE   B. FALSE   C. FALSE   D. FALSE   E. TRUE

Diathermy employs alternating current with a frequency of 1 MHz. The high current density at the intended site is what causes the tissue damage. Bipolar diathermy requires less power than unipolar and is used for delicate tissues eg in neurosurgery and ophthalmic surgery. Diathermy is not contraindicated if the patient has a pacemaker, but should be avoided if at all possible. Where unavoidable, bipolar diathermy is preferable to unipolar. If unipolar diathermy must be used then the plate should be placed as distant as possible from the pacemaker box. Diathermy can interfere with pacemaker function causing arrhythmias, triggering sensing and even reprogramming pacemakers. Unipolar diathermy can cause burns at the site of plate application if the area of contact with skin is reduced thus increasing current density. The plate should be carefully applied to clean skin and the site always inspected at the end of surgery.

Ref: Yentis Hirsch and Smith. Anaesthesia A to Z. Butterworth Heinemann.

ANSWER   11

A. TRUE   B. FALSE   C. FALSE   D. TRUE   E. TRUE

Hypertension is often present in patients with carotid stenosis. This shifts the autoregulation curve to the right. CBF does not vary directly with arterial oxygen content, hypoxia increases CBF and this response is enhanced in the presence of hypercarbia. CBF is related to $PaCO_2$ in a linear fashion and affected by cerebral metabolic rate, age, blood viscosity and temperature.

Ref: Miller. Anaesthesia 4th ed.

ANSWER   12

A. FALSE   B. FALSE   C. TRUE   D. FALSE   E. FALSE

AEPs involve the use of auditory stimuli (clicks) to generate an electric potential that can be measured over the auditory area of the brain. In order to cut out the effect of background potentials, including those produced by outside noises multiple responses are summed. Summation requires a number of consecutive signals so the AEP cannot be updated as frequently as every second. The AEP can be divided into three:

1. Brainstem AEP   (0-10 msec)   Posterior fossa surgery and hearing tests

2. Middle Latency AEP   (20-80 msec)   Depth of anesthesia monitoring

3. Late Cortical AEP   (>100 msec)   Conscious perception of sound.

Use of AEP as a monitor of depth of anaesthesia is felt to show great promise partly because it is mostly independent of the agent in use.

Ref: Kalkman, C.J. (1994) Monitoring the Central Nervous System. In: Sanford, T.J. (Ed.) Clinical Issues in Monitoring, pp. 173-196. Philadelphia: W B Saunders

ANSWER   13

A. FALSE   B. TRUE   C. TRUE   D. TRUE   E. FALSE

Cocaine may be taken by inhalation or sniffing as well as injection so needle marks may not be present in the chronic abuser of cocaine. Chronic use may result in serious cardiovascular and cerebral disease and lead to congenital anomalies. Hypertension, tachycardia, arrythmias, myocardial ischemia and infarction may result from cocaine use. Coronary artery disease does not seem to be induced in cocaine users and coronary vessel spasm is more the cause of ischaemia. Endocarditis may result from intravenous use. Pulmonary disease, apart from episodic pulmonary oedema from cardiovascular reasons, is not frequent. Central nervous system changes may lead to personality changes or more seriously to a seizure disorder which can also be induced on withdrawal. The Brompton Cocktail contains cocaine and so may prevent withdrawal problems in a user presenting for anaesthesia. Cardiovascular instability pre-operatively should be actively managed to prevent arrythmias or myocardial ischaemia occuring.

Ref. Katz. Anaesthesia and uncommon diseases. Chronic cocaine abuse.

ANSWER 14

A. FALSE   B. TRUE   C. TRUE   D. TRUE   E. TRUE

The 'Tec 6' is a non-variable bypass vapouriser allowing Desflurane to be used despite its high volatility and moderate potency. It's sump is heated to 39C at which its vapour pressure is twice atmospheric at sea level. This pressure provides the vapour circuit gas flow which is independent of the fresh gas flow. The 'Tec 6' requires manual adjustment for changes in atmospheric pressure to avoid a fall in absolute partial pressure of anaesthetic for a certain % setting at increased altitude. The working pressure of the vapouriser increases linearly with fresh gas flow to maintain an output of desflurane independent of fresh gas flow.

Ref: Miller. Anesthesia Church Livingstone. Desflurane, vapouriser.

ANSWER 15

A. FALSE   B. FALSE   C. TRUE   D. FALSE   E. FALSE

Status epilepticus should initially be treated with diazepam intravenously (in an emulsion form) or rectally. Phenytoin can be given as long as the rate does not exceed 50 mg/min in an adult and ECG monitoring is being used. Paraldehyde, clonazepam and chlormethiazole should be considered in addition to the above before thiopentone is considered. Phenytoin may increase plasma concentrations of phenobarbitone, and decrease those of clonazepam, carbamazepine, lamotrigine and valproate. Lamotrigine should be commenced at a low dose and increased every 2 weeks to reduce the incidence of side effects including Stevens-Johnson syndrome. Carbamazepine may cause hyponatraemia and this side effect has been used with beneficial effects in those with nephrogenic diabetes insipidus.

Ref: British National Formulary. 1996;32:203-213

ANSWER 16

A. FALSE   B. TRUE   C. FALSE   D. FALSE   E. FALSE

About 90% of PEs arise from the lower limbs and pelvis. Tachypnoea with shallow breaths is seen in 80% of patients and cyanosis is usually restricted to cases of massive PE. Tachycardia may relate to the site of obstruction and the onset of bradycardia is an ominous sign. It is imperative to maintain right heart filling pressures to perfuse the lungs and maintain right ventricular output therefore diuretics are contraindicated.

Ref: T.E. OH. Intensive Care Manual. Butterworths. 3rd Ed. Ch 26. Pulmonary embolism.

ANSWER 17

A. FALSE   B. FALSE   C. FALSE   D. TRUE   E. FALSE

Renal sodium wasting may result from :- Obstructive uropathy, Polycystic kidney disease, Addison's disease, congenital adrenal hyperplasia, unilateral renal artery stenosis resulting in the 'hyponatraemic hypertensive syndrome'.

Sodium retention may result from :- Nephrotic syndrome, glomerular disease e.g. diabetic nephropathy, chronic renal impairment from any cause, bilateral renal vascular disease.

Long term use of lithium may result in nephrogenic diabetes insipidus resulting in hypernatraemia if access to water is impaired.

Ref: Current Anaesthesia and Critical Care 1996; Vol 7, No 4: pg 176-181. Physiology and pathophysiology of fluids and electrolytes.

ANSWER 18

A. TRUE   B. TRUE   C. FALSE   D. FALSE   E. TRUE

The obesity in Cushings is typically central affecting the trunk. The associated proximal muscle wasting gives the so called "lemon on sticks " appearance. Muscle weakness can also occur without wasting and is caused by potassium depletion. Oligomenorrhoea is caused by the steroid excess. Depression affects 20% of patients.

Ref: Weatherall, Ledingham & Warrell. Oxford Textbook of Medicine. 2nd edition. vol 2. Section 10.70-10.71.

ANSWER 19

A. TRUE   B. FALSE   C. FALSE   D. TRUE   E. FALSE

Train of four = 4 supramaximal stimuli at 2Hz with a fixed pulse width of 0.2 ms. Force of contraction continues to slightly increase above the supramaximal threshold as a result of direct muscle stimulation. Therefore delivered current should ideally be 10-20% above the threshold. A train of four stimuli is used to detect fade on repetitive stimulation following non-depolarizing blockade. Fade is due to to non–depolarizer blockade of pre-junctional ACh receptors (which maintain ACH output with repetitive nerve stimulation). Post tetanic facilitation enables a response to occur when none was detectable following single twitches or TO4. The post tetanic count consists of a 5s 50Hz stimulus followed by a 3s pause and then single twitches at 1Hz. The number of detectable twitches is inversely related to intensity of block. Double burst stimulation = 3 x 50Hz stimuli separated by 0.75s.

ANSWER 20

A. TRUE   B. FALSE   C. FALSE   D. FALSE   E. TRUE

The aetiology of motor neurone disease and myasthenia gravis is unknown. Duchenne muscular dystrophy is an X linked recessive disorder. Acute intermittent porphyria presents in early adult life usually around the age of 30, women are affected more than men.

Ref: Kumar & Clark. Clinical Medicine. Balliere Tindall. Ch6, 18, 17

ANSWER 21

A. FALSE   B. TRUE   C. TRUE   D. FALSE   E. TRUE

Pneumonia is the commonest ICU infection. If the infection is present within 48 hrs of hospital admission, it is classified as a community acquired pneumonia. Principal pathogens (in decreasing incidence) are Streptococcus pneumoniae, Mycoplasma pneumoniae, Haemophilus influenzae and legionella species. The latter should be suspected if there has been recent travel abroad. Psittacosis is caught from birds and Q fever from farm animals. Recent influenzal infection should raise the possibility of Staphylococcus aureus infection and steroid therapy the possibility of tuberculosis. Ventilator acquired pneumonia has a mortality above 40%, the highest of which are in those due to Pseudomonas aeruginosa. Common pathogens include enterobacteriacae, P. aeruginosa and S. aureus although S. pneumoniae and H. influenzae are still encountered. Diagnosis of nosocomial pneumonia is difficult as pyrexia, pulmonary infiltrates and purulent ET secretions may be due to other causes. However, these signs and a fall in the PaO_2 are often used to diagnose the condition. ET aspirates correlate poorly with lower respiratory tract infection. Blood cultures are neither sensitive or specific in this condition. Quantitative culture using bronchoalveolar lavage may be useful.

Ref: Cooke RPD, Watson NA. Pneumonia in the ICU. British Journal of Intensive Care 1996;6: 126-133

ANSWER 22
A. FALSE   B. FALSE   C. TRUE   D. TRUE   E. FALSE

Mannitol and frusemide are equally effective and take 15-60 mins to exert their effect. However acute reduction is best produced by hyperventilation. Steroids should not be used in head injured patients.

Ref: Yentis, Hirsch,and Smith. Anaesthesia. Butterworths.

ANSWER 23
A. FALSE   B. FALSE   C. FALSE   D. FALSE   E. TRUE

The arbitrary definition of a massive transfusion is the replacement of a patient's total blood volume by stored allogenic blood in less than 24 hours or the acute administration of more than 1.5 times the estimated blood volume. The most common abnormality is an absolute thrombocytopaenia, but there is also a dilutional, as well as an absolute, fall in procoagulants and other essential components of the coagulation cascade. The platelet count falls in proportion to the volume of blood transfused; whereas plasma levels of factors V and VIII correlate poorly with transfusion volumes, and factor VII and fibrinogen levels are unrelated to transfusion volume. The normal haemostatic mechanism can function perfectly well with low procoagulant levels but diffuse microvascular bleeding appears to be mostly related to thrombocytopaenia and severe hypofibrinogenaemia. The most sensitive predictors of microvascular bleeding are a platelet count < 50,000/dl or a fibrinogen level < 0.5 g/l. For procoagulant levels to fall below 20% of their normal limits requires over two times blood volume replacement. The following has been suggested as the level of abnormal coagulation tests justifying treatment with FFP in the presence of generalized microvascular bleeding:-

Prothrombin time > 1.3 times control

Partial thromboplastin time > 1.3 times control

Thrombin time > 1.3 times control

Fibrinogen 100 mg/dl

Activated coagulation time > 150 seconds

Ref: Current Anaesthesia and Critical Care 1996; Vol 7, No 4: pg 192 - 196. The use and limitations of blood and blood products in resuscitation and intensive care.

ANSWER 24
A. TRUE   B. FALSE   C. FALSE   D. TRUE   E. TRUE

Lactic acid reacts with bicarbonate leading to CO_2 and lactate production. At a certain level of exercise the plasma lactate level rises sharply. This is at between 50-80% of maximal O_2 consumption. In an untrained person plasma lactate will rise at a lower level of exercise than in the trained. Glucose metabolism to lactate releases ATP at least twice as rapidly as mitochondrial metabolism and can optimally provide energy for 1.5 minutes of maximal muscle activity. After exercise 80% of lactate present is reconverted to glucose in the liver and restored in muscle and 20% is metabolised in the citric acid cycle. Filtered lactate is actively reabsorbed by the nephron to a transport maximum of 75 mg/min.

Ref: Paulev. Questions and answers in medical physiology. Chapter 39. Metabolism and exercise.

Ref: Guyton and Hall. Textbook of Medical Physiology. Chapter 84. Sports physiology. Chapter 72. Energetics and metabolic rate. Chapter 27. Urine formation by the kidney.

ANSWER 25

A. FALSE   B. FALSE   C. FALSE   D. TRUE   E. FALSE

Acute pancreatitis is most commonly due to gallstones or alcohol, although viral infections, drugs and trauma may provoke an episode. Most patients suffer epigastric pain, but all upper abdominal or chest pain should be viewed with suspicion. Pain may (rarely) be absent. Grey Turner's sign is flank bruising. Cullen's sign describes periumbilical bruising. Many sufferers recover without high dependency care, but in those with a severe attack, multiple organ dysfunction often occurs. Antibiotics are generally only prescribed when an infected necrotic pancreas is suspected, and in these cases the necrotic area should be debrided. Necrotic pancreatitis can be visualised with a contrast enhanced CT scan. Nasogastric suction, H_2 antagonists, TPN with 'bowel rest' and octreotide are often prescribed. The APACHE II severity scoring system is not able to predict individual mortality risk.

Ref: Kumar and Clark. Clinical Medicine (Third Edition). Bailliere Tindall. CH 5. Brady CE, Alvarez O. Acute pancreatitis. Current Opinion in Critical Care 1995;1:152-156

ANSWER 26

A. FALSE   B. FALSE   C. FALSE   D. FALSE   E. TRUE

The compositions of commonly used intravenous fluids must be known. 0.9% saline contains 154 mmol of sodium and chloride per litre. Albumin 4.5% has no calcium and gelofusine less than 0.4 mmol/l. Hence they can be infused before / after blood. Hartmann's solution has 131 mmol/l sodium, 5 mmol/l potassium, 2 mmol/l calcium and 111 mmol/l chloride. Dextrose saline 4% / 0.18%, contains 30 mmol/l of sodium and chloride.

Ref: Yentis, Hirsch, Smith. Anaesthesia A to Z. Butterworth Heinemann.

ANSWER 27

A. TRUE   B. FALSE   C. TRUE   D. FALSE   E. TRUE

Absolute humidity is defined as the mass of water in a volume of air. Relative humidity is defined as in the question and usually presented as a %. Humidification devices can be defined as active or passive; vapour or droplet producing; hot or cold and finally functioning in a breathing system or in the atmosphere. Theatre humidity should be around 60% as a compromise between discomfort (if too high) and the increased risk of explosion due to static electricity (if too low). Heat and moisture exchangers can achieve 70% humidification. A nebuliser works on the venturi or bernouille effect. For a bottle humidifier the water trap should be at least the same size as the humidifier bottle.

Ref: Ward. Anaesthetic equipment. Chapter 13. Humidifiers.
Craft & Upton: Key topics in anaesthesia. Humidification.

ANSWER 28

A. FALSE   B. FALSE   C. FALSE   D. TRUE   E. FALSE

Inspired gas is warmed and humidified in the nasopharynx and usually has a relative humidity of 90% and a temperature of 32–36°C. By the time gases have reached the alveoli they are fully saturated and at 37°C. Ciliary activity ceases above 41°C and slows down if relative humidity falls below 75% at 37°C. Humidification of inspired gases during mechanical ventilation reduces pulmonary complications and hypothermia. Methods include:

i) Saline drip - this is inefficient and dangerous and is not recommended.

ii) HMEs retain heat and moisture from the expired gases and return them during inspiration. They have become increasingly efficient and are now suitable for short term ventilation in many patients. They are not recommended for paediatrics or those with lung leaks as in these cases, much of the inspired gas does not pass through the HME on expiration.

iii) Cold water humidifiers - manage only 50% relative humidity and are not recommended in the critically ill.

iv) Hot water humidifiers - can be adjusted to administer 100% saturated gas at the endotracheal tube. However, tracheal scalding, condensation in circuits, inconsistent efficiency and infection (particularly Pseudomonas that multiplies in water reservoirs over 45°C in temperature) are disadvantages.

v) Nebulisers – gas driven, mechanical or ultrasonic which deliver micro-droplets. Ultrasonic nebulisers can cause overhydration, infection and an increase in airway resistance.

Ref: Oh. Intensive Care Manual. Butterworths. CH 24.

ANSWER 29

A. TRUE   B. TRUE   C. FALSE   D. FALSE   E. TRUE

Calcium antagonists selectively prevent ion entry through voltage-sensitive slow channels and are usually classified as

Class 1 antagonists (phenylalkylamines) - verapamil

Class 2 antagonists (dihydropyridines) - nifedipine

Class 3 antagonists (benzothiazepines) - diltiazem

Class 1 and 3 antagonists have significant effects on myocardial contractility and AV conduction whilst class 2 drugs predominantly affect peripheral blood vessels resulting in a reflex tachycardia. Anticholinesterase drugs result in bradycardias from their muscarinic effects and neostigmine has also been used in the management af supra-ventricular tachycardias. Hydralazine produces direct relaxation of smooth muscle by elevating intracellular cGMP. As there are no effects on the baroreceptors a reflex tachycardia results. Halothane increases vagal tone, depresses the SA node and its response to sympathetic stimulation and depresses AV conduction to produce a sinus bradycardia.

Ref: Calvey and Williams. Principles and Practice of Pharmacology for Anaesthetists. Blackwell. Chs 7, 9, 13, 14.

ANSWER 30

A. FALSE   B. TRUE   C. FALSE   D. TRUE   E. TRUE

Spinal shock after a spinal cord transection can last for days to weeks but has usually passed by approximately 3 weeks. Reflexes via the spinal cord below the injury lead to apparent sympathetic nervous system overactivity now unmodulated by higher inputs. These reflexes result from cutaneous or visceral stimulation and occur in 85% of patients. The resulting vasoconstriction can produce resting hypertension and hypertension in response to surgical and other stimuli even if the resting blood pressure is normal. The renin-angiotensin-aldosterone system is enhanced to help maintain blood pressure and patients may be very sensitive to angiotensin converting enzyme inhibitors. Vagal tone will be the only intact efferent in the baroreflex so bradycardia may be seen with changes in position, with a valsalva manoeuvre, or with increased intrathoracic pressure.

Ref: Priebe and Skarvan. Cardiovascular Physiology. Chapter 6. Cardiovascular control mechanisms.
Ref: Miller Anesthesia. Chapter 16. The autonomic nervous system.

ANSWER   31

A. FALSE   B. FALSE   C. TRUE   D. TRUE   E. FALSE

To successfully wean from mechanical ventilation, there must be a central drive, adequate respiratory muscle strength and a manageable load placed on these muscles. Lack of central drive may be due to any depressant medications, head or spinal cord injury or nervous system infection. Respiratory muscle weakness is caused by factors including infection, malnutrition, acidosis, hypercarbia, hypoxia, hypocalcaemia, hypomagnesaemia and hypophosphataemia.

Increased respiratory muscle workload may be caused by airways and circuits, hyperinflation, bronchconstriction, left ventricular failure and auto-PEEP. The latter also makes triggering of assist modes of ventilation more difficult. Before commencing, the patient should be adequately oxygenated- a PaO_2/FiO_2 ratio of greater than 250 should normally be present although this can be less in those with chronic lung disease or those with anatomical right to left shunts.

The f/Vt ratio during spontaneous ventilation (with CPAP as required) is a useful guide. After 5 minutes, if this is less than 80, success is likely. Above 105 failure is more likely and protracted weaning will probably be necessary. The maximum negative inspiratory pressure generated is useful to assess respiratory muscle strength. If it is less than -20 cmH$_2$O then severe weakness is present. If greater than -30 cmH$_2$O then as long as the lungs are compliant, spontaneous breathing should be possible. Most healthy adults acheive -100 cmH$_2$O.

Ref: Goldstone JC. Weaning from mechanical ventilation. Current Anaesthesia and Critical Care 1996;7:37-43

ANSWER   32

A. FALSE   B. TRUE   C. FALSE   D. TRUE   E. FALSE

Aldosterone causes sodium retention and potassium loss. In chronic renal failure hyponatraemia or hypernatraemia can occur. In acute renal failure fluid retention can lead to hyponatraemia. Hyperkalaemia can also occur and is an indication for dialysis. Hypopituitarism leads to a reduced secretion from the anterior pituitary gland and hence ACTH insufficiency and reduced cortisol. Mineralocorticoid production remains largely intact as this is predominantly stimulated by angiotensin II. Destruction of the entire adrenal cortex reduces glucocorticoids, mineralo-corticoids and sex steroids. As such hyponatraemia, hyperkalaemia and a raised urea result. Cushings results in excess cortisol which has some mineralocoticoid activity. This can lead to loss of potassium.

Ref: Kumar & Clark. Clinical Medicine. Balliere Tindall. Chapter 16.

ANSWER 33

A. FALSE   B. FALSE   C. FALSE   D. TRUE   E. TRUE

There are between 700 - 1500 deaths per annum in the UK from drowning. The incidence is 4 times higher in men than women and 2/3rds die in inland waters and 1/3rd in coastal waters. It is the 3rd commonest cause of death in chidren following RTAs and burns/smoke inhalation.

Outcome is dependent on the patient's state on arrival at hospital:

Awake & alert - 100% survival. Blunted consciousness - 2/37 died

		Children	Adults
Comatose on arrival	– normal recovery	44%	73%
	– persistent brain injury	17%	0%
	– died	39%	27%

Initial management revolves around the ABC of resuscitation and remember to record the patient's temerature because they're not dead until warm and dead. Patients with a GCS of 3, fixed dilated pupils and no cardiac output have been successfully resuscitated with no obvious neurological defecit if hypothermic. Patients need to be re-warmed and this should be done slowly with full monitoring on the ITU. Hypothermia results in an elevated SVR, cardiac dysfunction, makes VF difficult to treat if < 28-30°Centigrade and contributes to the profound acidosis that is often present (pH <7.1). Rapid re-warming may result in a rapid drop in the SVR leading to circulatory collapse in an already embarrassed heart. Steroids do not improve outcome and increase the secondary infection rate. There is no evidence that sodium bicarbonate raises arterial pH in drowning patients and it does not reverse intramyocardial acidosis. A rise in ICP is not immediate therefore ICP is not useful as a resuscitation parameter. Later a rise in ICP reflects the severity of brain injury and is therefore too late to affect outcome.

Ref: Critical Care Medicine. 1993; Vol 21: pg 368-73. Near Drowning
Ref: New England Journal of Medicine. 1993; Vol 328: pg 253-256. Drowning - a review

ANSWER 34

A. FALSE   B. FALSE   C. FALSE   D .TRUE   E. FALSE

A Sengstaken-Blakemore tube has 3 lumens; an oesophageal lumen, a gastric balloon lumen and a gastric aspiration lumen. It is passed via the nose or mouth, and once in the stomach the gastric balloon is inflated with about 250 ml of air. This should be done slowly, intermittently checking that the balloon pressure is no more than that when tested prior to insertion (to safeguard against oesophageal rupture). The tube is withdrawn until a resistance is felt, which is the balloon meeting the gasto-oesophageal junction. The tube is now placed on traction and this controls the bleeding as the varices are mainly fed from branches that cross this junction. The oesophageal balloon is less commonly inflated (25-35 mmHg) as the bleeding is often controlled by the gastro-oesophageal tamponade of the gastric balloon, and there is a risk of oesophageal rupture. This should be suggested by chest pain which calls for immediate oesophageal deflation. Pulmonary aspiration is a major risk due to the procedure and the condition of the patient it is being performed on. Endotracheal intubation should be carried out prior to insertion if it is felt there is risk of aspiration, and sedation should not be used to aid insertion.

Ref: Baskett, Dow, Nolan and Maull. Practical Procedures in Anesthesia and Critical Care. Mosby. Ch 3.

ANSWER 35

A. TRUE **B. FALSE** **C. TRUE** **D. FALSE** **E. TRUE**

The Kidneys receive 25% of the cardiac output and in health will present the proximal tubule with 180 L of filtrate per day. The oxygen consumption is 6 ml/100g/min, one of the highest in the body. The reabsorption of Na accounts for about half the O_2 consumption, which is directly related to the blood flow.

Ref: Scurr, Feldman & Soni: Scientific Foundations of Anaesthesia 4th ed.Heineman. p 410-11

ANSWER 36

A. FALSE **B. FALSE** **C. FALSE** **D. FALSE** **E. FALSE**

The rotameter is an example of a constant pressure, variable orifice flowmeter. If the pressure across a variable orifice remains constant the size of the orifice depends on the gas flow. At low flow rates, flow is a function of viscosity because the comparatively longer and narrower annulus between the float and the wall of the meter behaves like a tube i.e., is laminar. With higher flow rates the annulus is shorter and wider and behaves like an orifice so is density dependent. Readings are taking from the top of the bobbin in the rotameter. The pneumotaco-graph is a constant orifice, variable pressure flowmeter which senses the pressure difference across a fixed resistance using transducers. It is used to measure laminar flow. The Heidbrink flowmeter is a constant pressure, variable orifice flowmeter. Its bobbin is extended vertically to form a rod which functions in a similar way to the rotameter but does not rotate.

Ref: Yentis, Hirsch, Smith. Anaesthesia A to Z. Butterworth Heinemann.

ANSWER 37

A. TRUE **B. TRUE** **C. TRUE** **D. TRUE** **E. FALSE**

Using doppler ultrasound the incidence of venous air embolism is 50% in the patient sitting for a posterior fossa craniotomy compared to 10% if the patient is lying.

Ref: Craft & Upton. Key topics in Anaesthesia. Positioning the surgical patient.
Ref: Miller. Anesthesia. Patient positioning.

ANSWER 38

A. FALSE **B. FALSE** **C. TRUE** **D. FALSE** **E. TRUE**

Associations for peptic ulceration include smoking, blood group O, hypercalcaemia (and hence hyperparathyroidism), non-steroidal anti-inflammatory drugs as well as steroids. Duodenal ulcers usually occur in the 1st part of the duodenum (unless associated with Zollinger-Ellinson syndrome when they occur anywhere) and cause 'hunger' pain which is relieved by eating (c.f. gastric ulcer pain).

Ref: McLatchie. Oxford Handbook of Clinical Surgery. Oxford University Press.

ANSWER 39

A. FALSE **B. FALSE** **C. TRUE** **D. TRUE** **E. FALSE**

The apgar score was developed by an anaesthetist to ascertain the effects of anaesthetic agents on newly born infants. It measures 5 parameters, scored from 0-2, and should be measured at 1 and 5 minutes.

Ref: Yentis, Hirsch, and Smith. Anaesthesia A-Z. Butterworths. pp31-33

ANSWER 40

A. TRUE   B. FALSE   C. TRUE   D. TRUE   E. TRUE

Any process that significantly decreases FRC will lead to ventilatory failure. These should be thought of in sequence from lesions in the central nervous system (respiratory centre and upper motor neurone), spinal cord (anterior horn cells and lower motor neurone) and neuromuscular junction. Failure of respiratory muscles, chest wall or pleural integrity and inflammatory process within the lung. Lung compliance, the change in volume per unit pressure is decreased by the accumulation of extra lung water (pneumonia or LVF) and will increase the work of breathing. Ventilatory failure is defined as a pathological reduction of alveolar ventilation below the level required for the maintenance of normal arterial blood gas tensions. Mean normal arterial PCO_2 is 5.1kPa, the normal arterial oxygen content is dependent upon arterial PO_2 and haemoglobin concentration. Arterial PO_2 is affected by inspired oxygen concentration and shunting and the adequacy of ventilation is best defined by the arterial PCO_2.

Ref: Nunn JF. Applied Respiratory Physiology. Butterworths. Ch 20 pp379.

ANSWER 41

A. TRUE   B. FALSE   C. TRUE   D. FALSE   E. TRUE

2-12% of pregnancies are complicated by pre-eclampsia. It is a multi-system disorder, diagnosed after the 20th week of pregnancy by the triad of hypertension, peripheral oedema and protein-uria. Magnesium sulphate has a therapeutic range of 1.25-2.5 mmol/l.

Ref: Yentis, Hirsch, and Smith. Anaesthesia A-Z. Butterworths. pp366

ANSWER 42

A. FALSE   B. FALSE   C. TRUE   D. FALSE   E. FALSE

Myocardial contractility is not easily defined or measured. At a cellular level it is defined by the relationship between force and velocity of shortening. On the level of organ function, within the patient, dp/dt max. is sensitive to changes in preload and afterload so is a poor description of contractility. End systolic elastance (the inverse of compliance) is derived from the pressure volume loop of the ventricle and is a relatively load insensitive measure and so defines contractility well during changes in preload and afterload. An increase in contractility is defined by an increase in end-systolic elastance. An increase in contractility will increase myocardial oxygen consumption and so increase the likelihood of myocardial ischaemia. An increase in contractility in response to increased heart rate is described in the Bowditch effect. In response to an increase in afterload, contractility rises as defined by the Anrep effect.

Ref: Prys-Roberts & Brown. International Practice of Anaesthesia. Chapter 22. The heart - Myocardial metabolism and contraction - ventricular function.

ANSWER 43

A. FALSE   B. TRUE   C. FALSE   D. TRUE   E. TRUE

ACT can be measured in theatre using an automated system such as the Haemochron. 2ml of blood is mixed with 12mg of diatomaceous earth (a fine powder providing a large surface area for conversion of factor XII to XIIa). The end point occurs normally after 70-110 seconds when a clot is formed that prevents a magnetic rod in the bottle from maintaining the contacts between a switch in the base of the machine. The unit must be heated to 37°C to maintain reliable results. Hypothermic samples should be warmed or a correction applied. Haemodilution will also prolong the ACT. Although inter-patient response to heparin varies, individual dose responses are linear.

Ref: Miller RD. Anesthesia (Churchill Livingstone) Ch31.

ANSWER 44

A. FALSE   B. FALSE   C. TRUE   D. FALSE   E. TRUE

Fibreoptic bronchoscopy is useful for diagnosis, therapeutic lavage and perhaps tracheal intubation. It is usually of little use in the removal of inhaled foreign bodies where a rigid bronchoscope is used. It should be performed by someone with experience of the technique- usually a respiratory physician or intensivist. Obstruction of an endotracheal tube by the bronchoscope greatly increases the resistance to flow. Inspiration, being active, can often be manipulated using ventilator controls to maintain tidal volume. However, the use of bronchoscopic suction can reduce the alveolar ventilation. Tidal volume can be reduced by 75% at 21cmH$_2$O. Expiration, being passive, is also affected and expiratory flow hindered. PEEP values of 20 cmH$_2$O are possible. Bronchoalveolar lavage can cause severe hypoxaemia that persists for hours, and transbronchial biopsy may result in pneumothorax.

Ref: Morgan MDL. Fibreoptic bronchoscopy. Current Anaesthesia and Critical Care 1990;1:228-233.

ANSWER 45

A. TRUE   B. TRUE   C. FALSE   D. FALSE   E. TRUE

Coeliac plexus blockade is undertaken to denervate the foregut , interrupting nociceptive afferents from the pancreas, stomach, liver, and other viscera. It is usually performed under X-ray guidance, at T12-L1 via an angled posterolateral approach. Bilateral injections are performed to place anaesthetic / neurolytic agent anterolateral to the vertebral body in the thoracolumbar sympathetic chain. The abdominal aorta and inferior vena cava lie anterior to the chain. Although intravascular injection and spread to the lumbar somatic nerves is possible, postural hypotension is the most common complication due to visceral sympathetic blockade.

Ref: Miller RD. Anesthesia. Ch60. (Churchill Livingstone)

QUESTION 46

A. TRUE   B .FALSE   C. FALSE   D. TRUE   E. TRUE

Remifentanil. a pure mu receptor agonist, is a fentanyl derivative with an ester linkage. This leads to its rapid hydrolysis by non-specific tissue and plasma esterases – it is a poor substrate for pseudocholinesterase. Following cessation of an infusion designed to maintain a constant plasma concentration, the recovery from remifentanil is faster than that from alfentanil. It is equipotent with fentanyl, and 15-30 times more potent than alfentanil. As with other potent opioids, muscle rigidity can occur when large doses are infused intravenously.

Ref: Thompson JP, Rowbotham DJ. Remifentanil- an opioid for the 21st century. British Journal of Anaesthesia 1996;76:341-342

ANSWER 47

A. FALSE   B. TRUE   C. FALSE   D. FALSE   E. TRUE

Myasthenia gravis is characterized by fluctuating weakness and fatiguability. The patient is extremely sensitive to competitive non-depolarizing blockade due to a reduced receptor population. Sensitivity to suxamethonium is normal or reduced, however there have been numerous cases of Phase II block occuring even at doses of 0.5mg/kg. Anticholinesterase therapy potentiates vagal responses and inhibits pseudocholinesterase activity (which may reduce the hydrolysis of ester local anaesthetic agents).

Ref: Katz, Benumof, Kadis. Anesthesia and uncommon diseases. (WB Saunders)

ANSWER 48

A. TRUE   B. FALSE   C. FALSE   D. TRUE   E. TRUE

Hydroxyethyl starch is a synthetic macro molecular polymer manufactured by hydrolysing corn. It has a molecular weight ranging from 10,000 to over 1 million. The commonly used preparations are the hetastarches which are available in preparations with an average molecular weight of 200,000 and 450,000. The pentastarches have an average molecular weight of 250,000. Glomerular filtration is the major route of elimination and after 24 hours approximately 40% is left in the plasma. About 30% enters the RES, it is not known if this has any clinical significance. Large volumes lower factor VIII:C and may be clinically significant. The incidence of anaphylaxis is about 0.085% which is similar to the gelatins. Measured serum amylase may be elevated up to threefold following hydroxyethyl starch administration due to the delayed urinary excretion of amylase bound to the starch molecule.

Ref: Care of the Critically Ill 1995; Vol 11, No 3: pg 114-119. Crystalloids and colloids in the critically ill patient. British Journal of Hospital Medicine 1995; Vol 54, No 4: pg 155-160. The use of colloids in clinical practice.

ANSWER 49

A. FALSE   B. FALSE   C. TRUE   D. FALSE   E. FALSE

The trachea extends from C6 to opposite T4 or sometimes T5. It is supplied with blood from the inferior thyroid arteries. Lateral relations in the neck include the common carotid arteries, the lateral lobes of the thyroid, the inferior thyroid arteries and recurrent laryngeal nerves.

The trachea is composed of cartilaginous rings , fibrous membrane , muscular fibres , mucous membrane and glands. The muscular fibres are longitudinal and transverse. The longitudinal fibres are the most external and the transverse fibres (trachealis) are internal and form a thin layer between the ends of the cartilages and the posterior part of the trachea. The thyroid ima artery is a branch of the brachiocephalic artery but does not always exist.

Ref. Pick, Howden. Gray's Anatomy. Galley Press.

ANSWER 50

A. TRUE   B. TRUE   C. TRUE   D. TRUE   E . TRUE

Symptoms and signs which occur in a limb suffering arterial embolisation are pain, paraesthesia, paralysis, loss of distant pulses and pallor. Paraesthesia due to acute ischaemia of nerves will cause a loss of pin-prick and light touch sensation in a 'stocking' distribution.

Ref: Dunn & Rawlinson. Surgical Diagnosis and Management. Blackwell Scientific Publications.

ANSWER 51

A. FALSE   B. TRUE   C. TRUE   D. FALSE   E. FALSE

There are 4 basic modalities of ultrasound (M-mode, 2-D, Doppler, and Colourflow Doppler). Ultrasound is reflected back from tissue interfaces. The further away the tissue is the longer it takes for the reflected wave to return. When recorded against time this provides a typical M-mode display. Whilst useful for recording the timing of events this method has been superceded by the 2-D image for assessing structural detail. Resolution is acceptable down to 2.5mm. Doppler makes use of the change in frequency of sound reflected by moving objects. The modified Bernoulli equation allows calculation of the pressure difference across a stenotic valve (mmHg=4x[velocity in m/s]squared). Blood velocity in the normal heart is less than 1m/s. It will be increased by obstruction and stenosis. Colourflow Doppler superimposes a colour coded image of velocity on the two dimensional image allowing identification of high velocity jets, abnormal flow directions and shunts.

Ref: Kaufman L. Anaesthesia Review 10. (Churchill Livingstone). Ch1.

ANSWER 52

A. TRUE   B FALSE   C. FALSE   D. TRUE   E. TRUE

The adult allowances / kg body weight / 24 hours are :-

Water	30 ml
Energy	30 kcal (125 kJ)
Nitrogen	0.1-0.2 g
Glucose	3 g
Lipid	2 g
Sodium	1-2 mmol
Potassium	0.7-1.0 mmol
Calcium	0.1 mmol
Magnesium	0.1 mmol
Phosphorus	0.4 mmol

Ref: T.E. OH. Intensive Care Manual.Butterworths. Third Edition. Ch 82. Parenteral Nutrition

ANSWER 53

A. TRUE   B. TRUE   C. TRUE   D. TRUE   E. FALSE

Hypothyroidism is associated with oligomenorrhoea or menorrhagia or amenorrhoea. Bronchial carcinoma, especially small cell, may cause inappropriate ADH which leads to hyponatraemia.

A high arch palate is a commonly quoted feature of Marfans which may make intubation difficult, it is however rare. Aortic stenosis leads to a low fixed cardiac output which cannot respond to sudden needs to increase. Arrythmias such as VF can cause death. Hyperparathyroidism causes an increase in serum calcium, tetany is caused by hypocalcaemia.

Ref: Kumar & Clark. Clinical Medicine. Balliere Tindall. Chapter 16, 12, 11.

ANSWER   54

A. TRUE   B. FALSE   C. TRUE   D. TRUE   E. TRUE

Diarrhoea in critically ill patients prolongs hospital admission and places them at risk from noso-comial infections. It may be experienced by 34-41% of patients admitted to the ICU. The two commonest causes are due to medications or Clostridium difficile infection. Drugs associated with diarrhoea include antibiotics, magnesium containing antacids, digoxin, diuretics, antihy-pertensives, thyroid hormones and prokinetic agents. Clostridium difficile is responsible for pseudomembranous colitis and 20% of antibiotic associated colitis. Fulminant colitis and sepsis may follow. Clindamycin, penicillins, cephalosporins, neomycin and metronidazole are the antibiotics with the strongest association with C. difficile infection. Other causes include E. Coli, V. cholerae, other enteric pathogens and faecal impaction. Mesenteric ischaemia, whether due to mesenteric venous thrombosis, acute ischaemia or abdominal aortic aneurysm repair can cause diarrhoea, as can enteral nutrition. If the latter occurs, it may be due to a high osmolality feed, high rate of infusion or increased motility. A thorough review of medications, stool culture for pathogens (ova and parasites are extremely rare if diarrhoea develops more than 48 hrs after admission to hospital) and C. difficile toxin and rectal examination, supplemented where appropriate with sigmoidoscopy and radiological investigations will reveal the majority of causes. Diarrhoea due to enteral feed may require watering down or changing the feed, altering the infusion regime, or controversially, changing to parenteral nutrition.

Ref: O'Brien BL. Diarrhea in the critically ill. Current Opinion in Critical Care 1996;2:140-144

ANSWER   55

A. TRUE   B. FALSE   C. FALSE   D. FALSE   E. FALSE

Lyme disease can cause acute but reversible heart block due to its associated myocarditis.

Mobitz type 1 (Wenkebach) heart block is characterized by a progressively lengthening P-R interval, in Mobitz type 2 the P-R interval is constant prior to the non-conducted P wave. Following an inferior MI, second and third degree heart block is usually benign. Pacing is indi-cated only if the AV block is poorly tolerated and is resistant to atropine. The optimal pacemaker for sinus node disease is AAI ± R.

Ref: Current Anaesthesia and Critical Care 1995; Vol 6, No 3: pg 148-154. The diagnosis of brady-cardias and their management

ANSWER   56

A. FALSE   B. FALSE   C. TRUE   D. TRUE   E. TRUE

The radiation exposure during CT of head is similar to that of a conventional skull X-ray. Exposure values for personnel attending the patient are minimal but precautions are still recom-mended. Laryngoscopes are not magnetic but the batteries are and so plastic or paper coated ones must be used if a laryngoscope is to be used during magnetic resonance imaging. Myelography requires spinal lumbar puncture to inject the contrast material hence the patient must be prone. Anaesthesia may be required in the paediatric or uncooperative patient. Angiography to delineate the vasculature of the brain or spinal cord maybe improved by hyper-ventilation. Hypocarbia allows greater concentration of contrast material by slowing cerebral circulation and improves clarity by constricting cerebral vessels. Contrast media are radio-opaque iodine containing salts. Their injection may cause allergic reactions ranging from pruri-tus, burning on injection, skin rash, wheezing, dyspnoea, syncope or cardiovascular collapse.

Ref: Barash, Cullen, Stoelting. Clinical Anaesthesia. 2nd Edition. J.B. Lippincott Company.

ANSWER   57

A. FALSE   B. TRUE   C. FALSE   D. TRUE   E. FALSE

Anticoagulation is required prior to cannulation of the aorta or right atrium. This is most frequently achieved using heparin at a dose of 3mg or 300 units/kg. The degree of anticoagulation is checked using the activated clotting time which should be longer than 400-480 secs. Although systemic and myocardial cooling are commonly used for organ preservation there is some clinical trend towards warm bypass practice. If the aortic cannula is misplaced into the innominate artery or placed with its tip too far round the aortic arch one or both carotid pulses may be absent with parallel affects on cerebral perfusion. In the event of a significant arterial air embolism the patient should be placed in steep trendelenberg positon with compression of the carotids until hypothermic retrograde perfusion of the cerebral circulation via the superior vena cava cannula can be instituted with the aim of driving impacted air from the cerebral circulation. Nitrous oxide use should be stopped and the patient ventilated with 100% oxygen. Elective ventilation post-operatively would be appropriate.

Ref: Hensley FA Jnr. The practice of cardiac anaesthesia. Chapters 6 & 7.

ANSWER   58

A. FALSE   B. TRUE   C. FALSE   D. FALSE   E. FALSE

Trimetaphan blocks sympathetic and parasympathetic ganglia, releases histamine from mast cells and directly vasodilates blood vessels. It does not cross the blood brain barrier. Sodium nitroprusside causes arteriolar and venular dilatation by increasing nitric oxide levels (a mechanism shared with the nitrates but not with hydralazine which acts directly). It must be protected from the light as cyanide ions are otherwise formed. It can cause cyanide toxicity if the infusion rate is too high. This is exacerbated by renal failure as cyanide in the presence of thiosulphate is converted to thiocyanate which is renally excreted. Cyanide toxicity is treated with dicobalt edetate alone, or sodium nitrite followed by sodium thiosulphate. Dimercaprol is used for the treatment of heavy metal poisoning.

Ref: Calvey and Williams. Principles and Practice of Pharmacology for Anaesthetists. Blackwell Scientific Publications. Ch 13.

ANSWER   59

A. TRUE   B. FALSE   C. TRUE   D. TRUE   E. TRUE

Haemarthroses are often spontaneous and can lead to arthritic changes. The prothrombin time is sensitive to depletion of factors in the common and extrinsic coagulation pathway. In haemophilia A the intrinsic pathway is slowed so prothrombin time is normal. The bleeding time is a test for vascular disorders and platelet function. 0.4 mcg /kg of desmopressin intravenously may increase levels of factor VIII transiently in mild cases. Tranexamic acid (1g orally for adults) can also be given. Hepatitis B is due to numerous blood transfusions. It may eventually be possible to produce factor VIII by bioengineering methods.

Ref: Kumar & Clark. Clinical Medicine. Balliere Tindall. Chapter 6.

ANSWER 60

A. FALSE   B. FALSE   C. FALSE   D. FALSE   E. TRUE

Repeated doses of charcoal 50 gm initially then every 4 hours enhances the elimination of:

Aspirin

Carbamazepine

Dapsone

Phenobarbitone

Quinine

Theophylline

Ref: BNF 1996; No32: pg 20. Active elimination techniques (in Emergency treatment of poisoning pg 18-26)

ANSWER 61

A. TRUE   B. FALSE   C. FALSE   D. FALSE   E. FALSE

Standard deviation is the square root of the variance, the coefficient of variance is the mean divided by the standard deviation and will depend on the shape of the distribution. By definition 5% of normal values will be beyond 1.96 SD's and sample means are used to represent population means.

Ref: Yentis, Hirsch, and Smith. Anaesthesia A-Z. Butterworths.pp 418

ANSWER 62

A. TRUE   B. FALSE   C. FALSE   D. TRUE   E. FALSE

The mainstay of intra-operative neuromuscular monitoring is the train-of-four. On reversal of the blockade the return of a T4:T1 ratio of 0.75 suggests suitability for extubation, and correlates well with clinical signs. As the T4:T1 ratio is difficult to assess without a relaxograph, double burst stimulation was developed to allow more accurate consideration of the ratio. Post-tetanic count is used to monitor deep relaxation, when the train-of-four will not show any twitches. Normal neuromuscular function allows a sustained contraction when a supramaximal stimulus of 50Hz is supplied for 5 seconds. If the stimulus is of a higher frequency the fade may be seen with normal neuromuscular function. Tetanic stimuli (including post-tetanic count) can only be used once every 5 minutes.

Ref: Blunt, M.C. and Urquhart, J.C. (1997) The Anaesthesia Viva: Physics, Measurement, Clinical Anaesthesia, Anatomy and Safety, London: Greenwich Medical Media.

ANSWER 63

A. FALSE   B. TRUE   C. TRUE   D. TRUE   E. FALSE

Scoliosis may result in restrictive pulmonary deficit leading to pulmonary hypertension and right ventricular hypertrophy. Corrective surgery may be necessary to prevent further respiratory insufficiency or cardiovascular compromise. Harrington rods are used for surgical fixation, allowing distraction of vertebra using a ratchet. The 'wake-up' test involves intra-operative wakening to allow assessment of spinal cord function after the spine has been straightened. It is also used to assess cerebral function after basilar artery clipping. Recall is uncommon with careful anaesthetic technique.

Ref: Craft & Upton. Key Topics in Anaesthesia. Bios Scientific Publishers.

ANSWER 64

A. TRUE   B. TRUE   C. TRUE   D. FALSE   E. FALSE

The occurrence of gastroduodenal stress ulceration has reduced over the last few decades independently of specific prophylaxis, probably due to better management. The incidence of stress ulceration in the critically ill depends on the diagnostic criteria. Abnormal findings at endoscopy or a positive gastrocult may be present in over 70%. However, a 'significant bleed' i.e. haematemesis, coffee ground nasogastric aspirate, malaena or a haemoglobin drop of 2g/dl (complicated by cardiovacular instability or transfusion requirement) occurs in 5-20%.

Risk factors include CNS insults, hepatic, renal, respiratory or coagulation failure, burns, sepsis, shock, major surgery or trauma, organ transplantation and a history of peptic ulcer disease. Antacids are effective in reducing ulceration, but have been linked to an increased risk of nosocomial pneumonia. This may be due to increases in gastric intraluminal pH allowing bacterial colonization, but the volume of antacid and necessary presence of a nasogastric tube also result in increased risk of aspiration. H_2 antagonists are effective prophylactic agents. However, some (but not all) studies indicate a higher risk of nosocomial pneumonia. Sucralfate combines mucosal barrier protection, mucosal blood flow enhancement, stimulation of bicarbonate, mucus and prostaglandin secretion. Most studies indicate a lower incidence of bleeding compared with H_2 antagonists.

Ref: Levy MJ, DiPalma JA. Stress ulcer prophylaxis may not be for everyone. Current Opinion in Critical Care 1996;2:129-133

ANSWER 65

A. TRUE   B. TRUE   C. FALSE   D. FALSE   E. FALSE

The causes of confusion in ICU patients include;

   i) metabolic-urea, electrolyte, glucose and vitamin abnormalities.

   ii) cerebral hypoxia, hypercarbia, acidosis or hypertension.

   iii) drugs- administration and withdrawal (alcoholics may develop Wernicke's encephalopathy without rapid treatment)

   iv) infection or fever.

   v) pain.

   vi) psychiatric, endocrine or organic brain disease.

   vii) intracranial pathology.

   viii) cardiopulmonary bypass.

   ix) fat emboli.

   x) ICU psychosis- which should only be diagnosed when all others have been excluded.

Treatment is of the underlying cause, reassurance and communication (relatives and 'friendly faces' are often of great use), helping with sleep and occasionally restraint, sedation and psychiatric consultation.

Ref: HIllman and Bishop. Clinical Intensive Care. Cambridge University Press. CH 7.

ANSWER 66

A. TRUE   B. TRUE   C. FALSE   D. TRUE   E. FALSE

In acute appendicitis fever is not usually an early sign and where present it rarely rises above 38.5 degrees celsius. Urinalysis is usually normal though a few white and red cells may be present if the inflamed appendix is adherent to the ureter or bladder. Rovsing's sign is pain in the right iliac fossa produced by palpation in the left iliac fossa, and is positive in acute appendicitis. Anorexia is almost invariable, and the classical history is of colicky pain beginning centrally then moving into the right iliac fossa over several hours.

Ref: Forrest, Carter, Macleod. Principles and Practice of Surgery. Churchill Livingstone.

ANSWER 67

A. FALSE   B. TRUE   C. FALSE   D. FALSE   E. FALSE

Pseudo-obstruction is the development of symptoms of mechanical bowel obstruction related to (usually) the large bowel with no mechanical cause. It mostly affects elderly patients confined to bed with a recent history of illness or injury and is associated with underlying renal or cardiac disease, as well as disorders of water and/or electrolyte imbalance. Investigation (if required) is with water-soluble contrast enema (there is a risk of perforation) or colonoscopy, which can often decompress the distended colon. Laparotomy carries a high mortality.

Ref: McLatchie. Oxford Handbook of Clinical Surgery. Oxford University Press.

ANSWER 68

A. FALSE   B. FALSE   C. TRUE   D. FALSE   E. FALSE

SAH is usually due to rupture of an intracranial aneurysm. Sudden onset of headache, vomiting, unconsciousness,neck stiffness and focal signs are manifestations. CT scan usually confirms the diagnosis and often reveals the site and extent of the bleeding as well as complications such as oedema, infarction or hydrocephalus which can be responsible for a secondary deterioration and should be treated with ventricular drainage. Lumbar puncture should only be undertaken after CT scan to exclude raised intracranial pressure. Xanthochromia occurs after the blood has been present in the CSF for 6 hours. 50% of inpatients will die within 2 weeks if surgery is not performed. Rebleeding occurs in 15-20% and is most likely within the first day or after about 1 week. Vasospasm develops between days 5-14 and usually peaks at days 7-10. Cardiac dysfunction, hydrocephalus and convulsions may also occur. Treatment is general supportive care of a patient with raised ICP (including maintenance of an adequate cerebral perfusion pressure- beware reducing the blood pressure too drastically) If vasospasm occurs after (and in some centres before) the aneurysm is clipped, the cerebral perfusion pressure is artificially increased ('triple H' therapy- haemodilution, hypervolaemia and hypertension).

Ref: Hillman and Bishop. Clinical Intensive Care. Cambridge University Press. Ch 25.

ANSWER 69

A. TRUE   B. TRUE   C. TRUE   D. TRUE   E. TRUE

Sinus bradycardia due to activation of vagal reflexes during surgery may follow skin incision, stretching or dilatation of the anus, cervix, mesentary or bladder or pulling on the extra-ocular muscles. The stimulus should be stopped and if need be treatment with anti-cholinergics instituted.

Ref: Yentis, Hirsch and Smith. Anaesthesia A to Z. Butterworth Heinemann.

ANSWER 70

A. FALSE   B. FALSE   C. TRUE   D. FALSE   E. TRUE

Normal values are:-

CI 2.5 - 4 L/min/m^2

SVR 750 - 1500 dynes s cm^{-5}

DO$_2$I 550 - 750 ml/min/m^2

Ref: Soni. Anaesthesia and Intensive Care - Practical Procedures. Heinman Medical Books. Appendix 2

ANSWER 71

A. TRUE   B. FALSE   C. TRUE   D. FALSE   E. FALSE

Thoracotomy is indicated if over 1500ml or 200ml hour of blood is drained from a chest drain. The middle ribs (4 to 9) sustain the majority of rib fractures. The upper (1 to 3) ribs are protected by the scapula, humerus and clavicle. As such, their fracture indicates severe trauma. Fractures of the lower ribs (10 to 12) should raise suspicion of hepatosplenic injury. Fracture of the larynx is rare and characterised by hoarseness, subcutaneous emphysema and palpable fracture crepitus. Diaphragmatic rupture is more commonly diagnosed on the left because the liver obliterates the defect on the right. Suspected aortic injury should be evaluated by angiography. Computed tomography is unreliable.

Ref. Advanced Trauma Life Support Student Manual. American College of Surgeons.

ANSWER 72

A. TRUE   B. TRUE   C. TRUE   D. FALSE   E. FALSE

Colloids contain molecules which cannot cross a semipermeable membrane and are a suspension of molecules not a true solution as with crystalloids. They are divided into blood products and non-blood products, the latter including: starches, gelatins and dextrans which are sugars. Hapten pre-treatment is used for the dextrans. Hetastarch can produce plasma expansion for over 24 hours with pentastarch lasting rather less than 24 hours

Ref. Miller. Anesthesia. Artificial colloid solution therapy.
Ref. Yentis, Hirsch & Smith. Anaesthesia A to Z. Colloid.

ANSWER 73

A. FALSE   B. FALSE   C. TRUE   D. FALSE   E . TRUE

The right coronary artery arises from the anterior aortic sinus and the left from the posterior aortic sinus. The sinoatrial node is supplied by the right coronary artery which also supplies the atrioventricular node in 90% of hearts the remainder being supplied by the left. The left coronary artery bifurcates into the anterior descending and circumflex artery. These supply the anterior and lateral walls of the left ventricle and the interventricular septum. The right coronary artery gives rise to the posterior descending and a marginal artery. These supply the right ventricle, atrioventricular and sinoatrial nodes (as above) and posterior and inferior parts of the left ventricle. Inferior ischaemia (leads II. III, aVf) represents disease of the right coronary artery.

Ref. Barash, Cullen and Stoelting. Clinical Anaesthesia. 2nd edition. J.B. Lippincott Company.

ANSWER 74

A. TRUE   **B. FALSE**   **C. TRUE**   **D. FALSE**   **E. FALSE**

Normal cerebral blood flow is 50 ml/100gm/min. The effect of changes in CO_2 on cerebral blood flow are reduced over time as brain extracellular fluid bicarbonate levels adjust to normalise pH. The vascular response to hypoxia is not mediated via nitric oxide. The changes in cerebral blood flow are often gradual as mean arterial pressure goes above or below the autoregulatory limits and ischaemia will become apparent by symptoms only when mean arterial pressure is less than 60% of the lower autoregulatory limit.

Ref: Priebe and Skarvan. Cardiovascular Physiology. Chapter 7. Cerebral Circulation.

ANSWER 75

A. FALSE   **B. TRUE**   **C. TRUE**   **D. FALSE**   **E. FALSE**

The liver causes the right diaphragm to lie 2.5cm above the level of the left. In an AP portable chest X-ray the heart size is magnified. Even in a normal chest X-ray rotation will alter the radiographic density on each side. This can be assessed by determining whether the clavicular heads lie at an equal distance from the midline. The right hilum should lie at on the level of the lesser (horizontal) fissure while the left is about 1cm higher.

Ref: Corke & Jackson. Companion to Clinical Anaesthesia Exams. Churchill Livingstone. p 151

ANSWER 76

A. FALSE   **B. FALSE**   **C. TRUE**   **D. TRUE**   **E. TRUE**

The pleurae meet at the level of the second costal cartilage and descend to the fourth cartilage where the left deviates laterally. This occurs at the sixth cartilage for the right pleura. They cross the mid clavicular line at the eighth cartilage and the mid axillary line at the tenth. They terminate at the twelfth cartilage. The parietal pleura consists of cervical, mediastinal, costal and diaphragmatic types. The diaphragmatic portion lines the thoracic surface of the diaphragm and derives a nerve supply from the phrenic and lower 5 intercostal nerves. In the cervical region, the lung and pleura are closely adherent and have the same markings. At the root of the lung the pleura hang down inferiorly to form a cuff which allows for movement of the lung. The pleurae hang 2 intercostal spaces below the lung inferiorly. There are three spaces where the pleura are unguarded by ribs making them particularly vulnerable to puncture causing pneumothorax. These are at the right xiphisternal angle and below both sides of the twelfth thoracic vertebra between the ribs posteriorly.

Ref. Snell. Clinical Anatomy For Medical Students. Little Brown. Boston.

ANSWER 77

A. FALSE   **B. TRUE**   **C. FALSE**   **D. TRUE**   **E. TRUE**

Constriction of the major airways (eg asthma) reduces the FEV_1 more than the FVC. This results in a FEV_1 / FVC ratio less than the normal of 0.7. Restrictive lung disease (eg fibrosis) reduces the FVC and to a lesser extent the FEV_1. This results in a FEV_1 / FVC ratio of 0.7 or greater. Normally the FEV_1 is over 75% of the FVC. The maximum breathing capacity is measured by the subject breathing as deeply and as fast as they can over a 15 second period and measuring the volume of exhaled air. This correlates well with the FEV_1 but is more difficult to perform.

Ref: Corke, Jackson. Companion to Clinical Anaesthesia Exams. Churchill Livingstone.

ANSWER 78
A. FALSE   B. TRUE   C. FALSE   D. FALSE   E. TRUE

A short cuff causes readings to be too high whilst an overlapped long cuff does not cause error. Indirect measurement tends to overestimate at lower pressures and underestimates at higher pressures compared to direct measures. The oscillotonometer provides a good method for estimating systolic and mean pressures but not for diastolic pressures since a satisfactory end point for its estimation cannot be established. All oscillometric instuments (Dinamap, Accutorr) rely upon a regular cardiac cycle with no great difference between successive pulses, hence readings maybe inaccurate in atrial fibrillation. Continuous non invasive blood pressure measuring devices rely on a light emitting diode indicating the blood volume changes in a finger with systole and diastole. Using a servo system a cuff inflates and deflates to above systolic and then down to diastolic pressures. As soon as a pulse wave is sensed by the optical detector the servo increases the pressure so as to diminish the flow and so maintain a constant signal. Hence a pressure waveform identical to the intra-arterial waveform is produced and blood pressure measured.

Ref: Sykes, Vickers. Hull. Principles of Measurement and Monitoring in Anaesthesia and Intensive Care. 3rd Edition. Blackwell Scientific Publications.

ANSWER 79
A. TRUE   B. FALSE   C. FALSE   D. FALSE   E. FALSE

The sternal angle marks the junction between the manubrium sternum and the body of the sternum. The second costal cartilage joins the lateral margin of the sternum at this level. The highest point of the iliac crest lies at the level of the fourth lumbar vertebra (slightly inferior to the normal level of the umbilicus). The spinal anterior longitudinal ligament is a tough band that stretches from the atlas vertebra to the first piece of the sacrum . It is attached to the intervertebral discs and the vertebral bodies. The oesophagus together with the anterior and posterior vagal trunks and oesophageal branches of the left gastric artery pass through an oval hiatus in the muscular part of the diaphragm at the level of the tenth vertebra. The thyroid cartilage lies opposite the fourth cervical vertebra, the cricoid cartilage lies opposite the sixth.

Ref. Romanes. Cunninghams Manual of Practical Anatomy Vol. II English Language Book Society and Oxford University Press.

ANSWER 80
A. TRUE   B. FALSE   C. FALSE   D. TRUE   E. FALSE

A post-conceptual age of 60 weeks is sufficient to minimise the risk of post-operative apnoea as long as the neonate is not suffering from apnoeas anyway. No more prolonged starvation is needed than for other neonates and may be disadvantageous. The spinal cord ends higher than in adults and a block to the level of T10 will be adequate for inguinal hernia surgery. The risk of post-operative apnoea is reduced by spinal anaesthesia so long as no sedatives or opioids are administered.

Ref: Stehling L. Common problems in pediatric anesthesia. Chapter 14.

ANSWER   81

A. FALSE   **B. TRUE**   **C. TRUE**   **D. FALSE**   **E. FALSE**

In both the sympathetic and parasympathetic nervous systems all preganglionic neurones are cholinergic. The coronary vasculature is dilated (beta2), and constricted (alpha1), by the adrenergic system. In the presence of an intact endothelium parasympathetic stimulation leads to a dilatation via the actions of nitric oxide. The paired stellate ganglia send postganglionic fibres to the heart. Stimulation via the right leads to increased heart rate while via the left leads to increased contractility. Resting sympathetic tone maintains a greater contractile state compared to the denervated heart. Alpha2 mediated negative feedback functions by reducing intra-cellular levels of cAMP. Circulating catecholamines have a t1/2 of less than 20 seconds, then being taken up by tissues and inactivated in the liver and vascular endothelium. This allows very rapid adjustments in the effects of sympathetic stimulation.

Ref: Priebe and Skarvan. Cardiovascular Physiology. Chapter 6. Cardiovascular control mechanisms.
Ref: Paulev. Questions and answers in medical physiology. Chapter 15. The autonomic nervous system.

ANSWER   82

A. FALSE   **B. FALSE**   **C. FALSE**   **D. TRUE**   **E. TRUE**

Transcutaneous Electrical Nerve Stimulation (TENS) involves stimulating large sensory nerve fibres (A-beta) in order to inhibit the transmission of impulses from unmyelinated C fibres in the dorsal horn of the spinal cord. Impulses should be 0-50mA, 0-100Hz with a pulse width of 0.1-0.5ms. TENS is potentially effective for any localised somatic or neurogenic pain provided paraesthesia can be generated in the region of the pain. Visceral pain such as angina has been successfully treated with the technique. It may be used for acute pain (labour, post operative pain) or chronic pain (peripheral neuralgia, post-herpetic neuralgia, chronic back pain, etc). There are a number of studies showing TENS to be better than placebo, however one of the major problems with its use is the development of tolerance to the analgesic effect, and changes in the pattern and type of stimuli may help this.

Ref: Woolf, C.J. and Thompson, J.W. (1994) Stimulation fibre-induced analgesia: transcutaneous electrical nerve stimulation (TENS) and vibration. In: Wall, P.D. and Melzack, R. (Eds.) Textbook of Pain, 3rd edn. pp. 1191-1208. Edinburgh: Churchill Livingstone

ANSWER   83

A. FALSE   **B. FALSE**   **C. FALSE**   **D. TRUE**   **E. FALSE**

During genito-urinary procedures, patients with a heart valve lesion, septal defect, patent ductus, prosthetic valve or a previous history of endocarditis should receive a combination of amoxycillin and gentamicin. If they are penicillin sensitive or have received more than one dose of a penicillin within the previous month, alternatives are vancomycin and gentamicin, or teicoplanin and gentamicin. Organisms responsible for infected urine should also be covered. For a patient with a previous history of endocarditis undergoing a procedure that warrants prophylaxis, the guidelines are similar to those above. Another alternative in those undergoing dental or upper respiratory tract procedures is clindamycin. Prophylaxis for obstetric procedures is only required for those with prosthetic valves or a history of endocarditis.

Rifampicin, or possibly ciprofloxacin or ceftriaxone should be given to close contacts to prevent secondary cases of meningococcal meningitis. In addition to cover against H. Influenzae in a child following splenectomy, pneumococcal infection prophylaxis is necessary.

Ref: British National Formulary 1996;32:228-229

ANSWER 84

A. FALSE   B. FALSE   C. TRUE   D. TRUE   E. FALSE

SDD is an antibiotic regimen which aims to reduce the incidence of nosocomial infection in critically ill patients by selective destruction of the pathogenic gut micro-organisms, in particular gram-negative organisms. The anaerobic gut flora are important to prevent overgrowth of gram-negative enteric bacilli therefore metronidazole is specifically contraindicated in those patients on the SDD regimen. Clinical trials have demonstrated that SDD significantly reduces the incidence of of nosocomial respiratory infections. However, except in trauma patients, SDD has not demonstrated any improvement in mortality. The regimen as described by Stoutenbeck et al in 1984 involves:-

1. Amphotericin suspension 200 mg, Colomycin elixir 1,000,000 units, Tobramycin 80 mg Administered by mouth or nasogastric tube 6 hourly

2. Oral paste or gel containing 2% of each antibiotic 6 hourly

3. Cefotaxime 1 gm iv 8 hourly for 4 days

Ref: Current Anaesthesia and Critical Care. Churchill Livingstone. 1996. Vol 7, No 2, pg77 - 80. Selective decontamination of the gut: an update.

ANSWER 85

A. TRUE   B. TRUE   C. FALSE   D. TRUE   E. TRUE

This is watery or bloody diarrhoea associated with broad-spectrum antibiotic therapy. It is caused by overgrowth of Clostridium difficile and usually presents 5-10 days after commencing antibiotic therapy. It is treated with oral metronidazole or oral vancomycin (which is not absorbed from the GI tract, hence levels are irrelevant), but is recurrent in up to 30% of cases.

Ref: McLatchie. Oxford Handbook of Clinical Surgery. Oxford University Press.

ANSWER 86

A. FALSE   B. TRUE   C. FALSE   D. FALSE   E. TRUE

Adenocarcinomas are the commonest carcinoma associated with asbestosis and occupational factors such as exposure to arsenic, chromium, iron oxide, petroleum products, coal tar and radiation. It is more common in women, the elderly and in the Far East. Enophthalmos, pupillary constriction, ptosis and loss of sweating is Horners syndrome. This can occur if an apical carcinoma invades the sympathetic ganglion. Chest X-rays are relatively insensitive at picking up carcinomas and the tumour needs to be over 1cm in size to be reliably recognised. Prednisolone, up to 15mg daily, maybe used to improve appetite in the terminal care of patients with bronchial carcinoma.

Ref: Kumar & Clark. Clinical Medicine. Balliere Tindall. Chapter 12

ANSWER 87

A. TRUE   B. FALSE   C. TRUE   D. FALSE   E. TRUE

Irrigation solutions need to be non electrolyte , heat stable and nonhaemolytic. Hypotonic glycine is used for its optical properties. The maximum recommended height for suspension of the irrigation bag is 60cm above the patient. TURP syndrome is more common when the prostate capsule is opened and in those patients with poor myocardial reserve, and following long operations. It may present as blindness due to cortical oedema.

Ref: Agin C. Anaesthesia for transurethral prostate surgery. Int Anes Clinics 31.pp25-46

ANSWER 88

A. TRUE   B. FALSE   C. FALSE   D. FALSE   E. TRUE

Prior to pneumonectomy there are several predictors of functional outcome. Arterial blood gases and simple spirometry are useful baseline tests: MBC and FEV1 should both be greater than 50% predicted and an arterial $PaCO_2$ should be <45 mmHg. If any of these results are out of range then ventilation and perfusion scans should be performed. If these are out of acceptable limits and surgery still considered then invasive unilateral pulmonary arterial occlusion with and without exercise should be examined to determine if surgery is feasible. Prognosis is worse after the age of 75 and is not affected by position.

Ref: Miller RD. Anesthesia 3rd ed. Churchill Livingstone. Ch50 pp 1520

ANSWER 89

A. FALSE   B. TRUE   C. TRUE   D. TRUE   E. TRUE

$SvO_2 = SaO_2 - (VO_2 / 1.31 \times [Hb] \times CO)$

It is therefore increased by: Increasing SaO_2, reduction in oxygen uptake (VO_2), and increases in haemoglobin and cardiac output. Haemorrhage causes a fall in haemoglobin and cardiac output, and an infusion of adrenaline causes an increase in cardiac output. The pulmonary artery catheter will give inaccurate measurements of mixed venous saturation if wedged or if mitral regurgitation causes a backflow of oxygenated blood onto the tip of the catheter.

Ref: Moon, R.E. and Camporesi, E.M. (1990) Respiratory Monitoring. In: Miller, R.D. (Ed.) Anesthesia, 3rd edn. pp. 1129-1163. New York: Churchill Livingstone

ANSWER 90

A. FALSE   B. FALSE   C. TRUE   D. FALSE   E. FALSE

Colonic carcinoma is almost always adenocarcinoma. Duke's B tumours involve spread through the bowel wall but not the lymph nodes. 90% are operable even if only for palliation. 25% present as emergencies with either obstruction, bleeding or perforation and peritonitis. Transfusion of whole blood increases tumour recurrence (thought to be related to plasma components initiating an adverse immunological reaction) and should be avoided. Red cell concentrate is preferable.

Ref: McLatchie. Oxford Handbook of Clinical Surgery. Oxford University Press.

Exam 2

QUESTION 1

In myocardial infarction

A. Serum AST falls after CK and LDH
B. The incidence in females aged 20 - 64 is 3.5 per 1000 in Western communities
C. Treatment with streptokinase can cause hypotension
D. The patient's temperature can be raised
E. Atrial arrythmmias are the commonest form of arrythmia

QUESTION 2

Spontaneous pneumothorax

A. May lead to surgical emphysema
B. Is typical in obese patients
C. Is commonly associated with emphysema
D. Oxygen is the therapy of choice
E. Is painful

QUESTION 3

Concerning jaundice

A. Dark urine and pale stool are the hallmarks of obstructive jaundice
B. Is clinically detectable when the plasma total bilirubin exceeds 20 micromols/l
C. Pain is not a feature of carcinoma of the head of pancreas
D. Jaundice may complicate treatment with chlorpromazine
E. Is an early feature in cirrhosis of the liver

QUESTION 4

Hyperthyroidism is associated with

A. Somnolence
B. Hypercalcaemia
C. Diabetes mellitus
D. Pretibial myxoedema
E. Delayed tendon reflexes

QUESTION 5

The following are features of hypercalcaemia

A. Prolonged QT interval on ECG
B. Diarrhoea
C. Coma
D. A positive Trousseau's sign
E. Cataracts

QUESTION 6

Concerning phaeochromocytoma

A. Tumours all arise in the adrenal medulla
B. Diarrhoea and constipation are features
C. Glycosuria is present
D. Signs and symptoms are usually sustained
E. Urinary vanillylmandelic acid is elevated

QUESTION 7

In carbon monoxide poisoning the following are common

A. Cyanosis
B. Angina
C. Nausea and vomiting
D. Convulsions
E. A normal oxygen saturation on pulse oximetry

QUESTION 8

In chronic constrictive pericarditis

A. Pedal oedema is present
B. The heart sounds are quiet
C. Medical treatment with diuretics is indicated
D. Prominent ascites may occur
E. SVC obstruction is a feature

QUESTION 9

Percussion note is dulled over the following lesions

A. Pneumothorax
B. Pleural effusion
C. Pulmonary TB
D. Consolidation secondary to infection
E. Oedema secondary to heart failure

QUESTION 10

The following conditions are associated with a haemoglobin concentration of 7 g/dl and a mean corpuscular volume of 70 fl

A. Iron deficiency anaemia

B. Acute blood loss

C. Folate deficiency

D. Renal failure

E. Thalassaemia

QUESTION 11

During laparoscopic surgery

A. A 30% increase in arterial CO_2 may occur

B. Intra-abdominal insufflation of nitrogen at the end of the procedure may cause shoulder pain

C. Venous return is impaired

D. The functional residual capacity rises

E. Venous return is enhanced

QUESTION 12

Concerning pre-operative obstructive jaundice

A. Raised alkaline phosphatase suggests extra-hepatic obstruction

B. Vitamin K should be administered

C. Plasma bilirubin > 100 umol/l carries a poor prognosis

D. Haematocrit < 30% carries a poor prognosis

E. Extra-dural anaesthesia is contraindicated

QUESTION 13

The following represent major risk factors for deep venous thrombosis (DVT)

A. Myeloma

B. Age < 40 years

C. Paraplegia

D. The oral contraceptive mini-pill

E. Protein C deficiency

QUESTION   14

In the patient with a spinal injury

A. Priapism suggests cervical cord injury

B. Hypotension and bradycardia maybe present in the absence of hypovolaemia

C. Corticospinal tract injury occurs in damage to the anterolateral aspect of the cord

D. Spinal shock is characterised by spasticity followed by flaccidity after several days to weeks

E. Most vertebral body fractures at T4 are unstable

QUESTION 15

Tracheo-oesophageal fistula

A. Is diagnosed with the use of radio-opaque contrast media

B. Is commonly associated with oesophageal atresia

C. Tracheomalacia is a complication after surgery

D. Surgery is performed via left thoracotomy

E. Occurs more commonly in males

QUESTION 16

The following are associated with an increased risk of malignant change

A. Ulcerative colitis

B. Crohns disease

C. Familial polyposis coli

D. Plummer-Vinson syndrome

E. Adenomatous villi

QUESTION 17

Concerning coronary artery bypass grafting

A. Mortality is higher in males

B. Internal mammary artery grafts give prolonged patency over saphenous vein grafts

C. Life expectancy is improved in the absence of angina

D. Life expectancy is improved in triple vessel disease

E. Mortality is < 1% for two grafts

QUESTION 18

Acute appendicitis

A. Presents with diarrhoea

B. Is the commonest cause of an acute abdomen in the UK

C. Causes a lymphocytosis

D. Differential diagnosis includes basal pneumonia

E. Causes microscopic haematuria

QUESTION 19

When acrylic cement is used for fixation of orthopaedic prostheses

A. Fat embolism may result

B. A temperature of 90 degrees celsius may be generated locally as it hardens

C. Cardiovascular collapse is lessened by saline irrigation of the bone cavity prior to cement insertion

D. The risk of hypotension is reduced by applying the cement by hand

E. Peripheral vasoconstriction occurs

QUESTION 20

Malignant tumours of the following organs commonly metastasise to brain

A. Pancreas

B. Liver

C. Uterus

D. Ovary

E. Lung

QUESTION 21

When used for premedication

A. Midazolam can be administered intramuscularly

B. Cyclizine increases lower oesophageal sphincter tone

C. Hyoscine has no effect on the incidence of awareness

D. Rectal thiopentone (40mg/kg) produces predictable and reliable sedation

E. The effect of metoclopramide on gastric motility is antagonized by atropine

QUESTION 22

Prolonged neuromuscular blockade following the use of suxamethonium

A. Is more likely to be due to the atypical gene rather than the fluoride gene

B. Is always due to inherited abnormalities of plasma cholinesterase

C. Should be treated with an anticholinesterase if a dual block is present

D. May be due to hypothyroidism

E. A patient heterozygous for the atypical gene will have a dibucaine number of between 50–80

QUESTION 23

Concerning Mivacurium

A. It consists of ten stereoisomers, as supplied clinically
B. The cis-trans isomer has a low plasma clearance
C. In patients with cirrhosis the plasma clearance of the cis-cis isomer is decreased
D. Its duration of action varies inversely with plasma cholinesterase activity
E. It should not be used in patients with myasthenia gravis

QUESTION 24

When choosing a route for drug administration

A. Fentanyl can be administered intranasally, but the equianalgesic dose required is approximately 5 times the iv dose
B. Midazolam is licensed for oral administration
C. Drugs to be given by the transdermal route must have lipid and aqueous solubility
D. Oral transmucosal drug delivery avoids hepatic first-pass metabolism
E. Transdermal scopolamine patches are recommended to be placed on the thigh

QUESTION 25

In the drug treatment of schizophrenia

A. Chlorpromazine is more likely to cause sedation than haloperidol when given orally
B. Movement disorders are due to D_1 receptor blockade
C. Oral haloperidol may cause movement disorders
D. Dystonias can be treated with orphenadrine
E. Anticholinergic side effects are rarely problematical

QUESTION 26

The following benzodiazepines have significant active metabolites

A. Oxazepam
B. Diazepam
C. Triazolam
D. Chlordiazepoxide
E. Lorazepam

QUESTION 27

Pulmonary fibrosis can be caused by

A. Bretylium
B. Paraquat
C. Prednisolone
D. Bleomycin
E. Chloroquine

QUESTION 28

Nitric oxide

A. Is synthesised in vascular endothelium from L-citrulline
B. Is synthesised largely by an enzyme independent process in response to changes in pulsatile flow
C. Is important in maintaining basal tone in coronary vessels
D. Produces its effects on vascular tone by a direct effect on Ca^{++} channels in resistance vessels
E. Has a half life of 10 minutes in vivo

QUESTION 29

During intermittent positive pressure ventilation

A. Mean intrathoracic pressure will be lower than during spontaneous breathing
B. Right ventricular filling rises secondary to raised pulmonary vascular resistance
C. Regional anaesthesia may affect cardiac output
D. PEEP will reinflate collapsed alveoli
E. Left ventricular workload may decrease

QUESTION 30

Gastrointestinal secretions are affected by

A. Atropine as a result increased vagal tone
B. Cimetidine secondary to proton pump inhibition
C. Antacids
D. The presence of osmotic particles
E. Diuretics

QUESTION 31

Concerning bilirubin and its metabolism

A. Bilirubin is produced in macrophages by reduction of biliverdin
B. Bilirubin is transported to the liver in uncombined form
C. 10% of bilirubin entering the hepatocytes undergoes sulphonation
D. 50% of urobilinogen absorbed from the gut is renally excreted
E. In biliary obstruction conjugated bilirubin will not appear in the urine

QUESTION 32

During apnoea at rest the PaCO$_2$ rises by

A. Displacement of alveolar oxygen
B. 5 kPa per minute
C. 10 kPa per minute
D. Equilibration with PvCO$_2$
E. Equilibration with PACO$_2$

QUESTION 33

Diastolic filling of the left ventricle

A. Is aided by a modest tachycardia when the left ventricle is hypertrophied
B. Occurs mainly in later diastole, including the time of atrial systole
C. Active relaxation is improved by sympathetic stimulation in the setting of a steady heart rate
D. Is most commonly disturbed by hypertensive cardiac disease
E. Can be represented by a constant of ventricular stiffness

QUESTION 34

In the splanchnic and renal circulations

A. Hepatic blood flow in an adult is normally 1000 ml/min
B. The capacitance blood vessels hold 30% of the total blood volume
C. Beta2 receptors in the splanchnic circulation lead to vasodilatation
D. Renal blood flow is autoregulated between perfusion pressure limits of 75 to 180 mmHg
E. Intrarenal prostaglandin production helps reduce renal ischaemia during shock

QUESTION 35

Acidosis

A. Is different from acidaemia
B. Resulting from metabolic causes is due to a raised PaCO$_2$
C. If metabolic in nature leads to hyperventilation
D. Results in a higher than normal plasma pH
E. Should be treated with bicarbonate therapy

QUESTION 36

Within the kidney

- **A.** The afferent and efferent arterioles provide a higher resistance to blood flow than any other organ
- **B.** The cells of the juxtaglomerular apparatus are found in the efferent arteriole
- **C.** Angiotensin II produces a fall in blood flow
- **D.** The plasma oncotic pressure rises throughout the length of the glomerular capillary
- **E.** Glomerular capillary permeabilty is lower than in other organs

QUESTION 37

The extradural space can contain

- **A.** Fat
- **B.** Spinal nerve roots
- **C.** Lymphatics
- **D.** Batson's plexus
- **E.** Connective tissue

QUESTION 38

Concerning the intercostal space

- **A.** The anterior intercostal arteries emerge from the internal thoracic artery
- **B.** The intercostal nerves are the posterior primary rami of the thoracic spinal nerves
- **C.** The intercostal nerves lie superior to the arteries in the costal groove
- **D.** The intercostal nerves and vessels lie between the internal and external intercostal muscles
- **E.** The intercostal nerves are motor and sensory

QUESTION 39

The stellate ganglion

- **A.** Is present in all subjects
- **B.** Lies on the flat lateral border of T2
- **C.** When blocked can provide pain relief for herpes zoster infections
- **D.** Chassaignac's tubercle is a landmark when preparing to block it
- **E.** Is formed by the fusion of the first 2 thoracic sympathetic ganglia

QUESTION 40

The first rib

A. Is crossed superiorly by the subclavian artery
B. Has an under surface with grooves for muscular attachment
C. Is the most curved rib
D. Is a false rib
E. Has no angle

QUESTION 41

The Exercise ECG

A. Is "positive" if the patient concludes the test without developing angina
B. Has a false-positive rate of up to 25%
C. Is diagnostic of ischaemia if the patient develops pain and 2mm down sloping ST depression
D. Down sloping ST segment depression is more significant than up sloping depression
E. Is more sensitive if a treadmill protocol is used rather than simple step tests

QUESTION 42

Direct arterial pressure measurement

A. Critical damping is ideal to ensure an optimum trace
B. The measurement system should have a natural frequency of about 100Hz
C. A continuous flush device delivers 15 ml/hr through the cannula
D. Rate of rise of LV pressure is most accurately demonstrated by a system with a high natural frequency
E. Allows beat-by-beat measurement

QUESTION 43

Concerning blood gas analysis

A. The hydrogen ion measurement electrode is maintained at 37°C
B. Response time of the carbon dioxide electrode is slower than the hydrogen ion measurement system
C. The hydrogen ion measurement system consists of a silver / silver chloride electrode in contact with a bicarbonate buffer
D. The Severinghaus carbon dioxide electrode contains a glass electrode sensitive to carbon dioxide
E. The oxygen electrode consists of a platinum cathode in direct contact with blood for analysis

QUESTION 44

The following cause errors in the measurement of oxygen saturation by pulse oximetry

A. Haemoglobin S
B. Methylene blue
C. Severe anaemia
D. Acute severe hypoxia
E. Jaundice

QUESTION 45

The following methods can be used to measure carbon dioxide

A. Interferometer
B. Polargraphic cell
C. Chromatography
D. Adsorbtion onto rubber strips
E. Infra-red absorption

QUESTION 46

Pulmonary artery catheter information

A. Calculation of left ventricular stroke work requires the mean arterial pressure
B. A high systemic vascular resistance is suggestive of sepsis
C. Indexing of systemic vascular resistance (SVRI) is achieved by dividing the SVR by the body surface area
D. The PVR is a poor indicator of the resistance of the pulmonary vasculature to blood flow
E. The PA systolic and diastolic pressures are on average 30% inaccurate at high heart rates

QUESTION 47

The following lead to inaccuracies when determining cardiac output by thermodilution

A. Injectate volume less than 10 ml
B. Tricuspid incompetence
C. Intracardiac shunts
D. Pulmonary artery thermistor thrombus
E. Warmed injectate fluid

QUESTION 48

The following are features of depolarising blockade

A. Tetanic fade
B. Post-tetanic potentiation
C. Antagonism by anticholinesterases
D. Potentiation by pancuronium
E. Progression to dual blockade

QUESTION 49

Activated coagulation time

A. Is measured by the 'Hemochron'
B. Is normally maintained at x3 normal ratio for cardiopulmonary bypass
C. Is measured following in vitro factor X activation
D. Is measured at 20°C
E. Is prolonged by haemodilution

QUESTION 50

Electroencephalogram (EEG)

A. Measures the electrical activity of the outer 2-3 mm of the cerebral cortex
B. In the awake adult the dominant EEG frequency is normally alpha
C. Opioids have little effect on the EEG
D. Enflurane causes loss of the dominant frequency, increase in beta activity and then high-voltage delta and theta activity
E. EEG may be used to monitor cerebral ischaemia

QUESTION 51

During the course of septicaemia

A. Cardiac index increases initially
B. Hypothermia is a feature
C. Nitric oxide production relaxes vascular smooth muscle via cyclic adenine monophosphate
D. Cardiac dysrhythmias occur in 40% of patients
E. Thrombocytosis is a common finding

QUESTION 52

When interpreting liver function tests

A. AST is more liver specific than ALT
B. AST is more sensitive than ALT to liver damage
C. Reduction in albumin concentration is more likely to be as a result of protein catabolism than decreased synthesis
D. ALP increases occur with biliary tract dysfunction
E. Only coagulation factors II, VII, IX and X are synthesised in the liver

QUESTION 53

The APACHE II severity of disease classification

A. Does not assign points according to age
B. Should not be used to predict individual mortality risk
C. Combines the APACHE II score and diagnostic category to predict group mortality
D. Does not require a serum urea level to compute a score
E. Can be used for the patients first 24 hours in the intensive care unit

QUESTION 54

Important complications of total parenteral nutrition (TPN) include

A. Sepsis
B. Metabolic alkalosis
C. Rebound hyperglycaemia on sudden discontinuation
D. Hyperosmolar dehydration syndrome
E. Zinc deficiency

QUESTION 55

Concerning brain stem death and organ donation

A. If a patient carries a signed donor card there is a legal requirement to establish lack of objection from next of kin
B. Jehovah's Witnesses as a religious group do not object to donating or receiving organs
C. Doll's eyes reflex must be absent for the criteria to be fulfilled
D. The apnoea test requires the $PaCO_2$ to exceed 6.65kPa (50mmHg) to be positive, following appropriate oxygenation
E. Testing should be delayed for at least 24 hours following a hypoxic cardiac arrest

QUESTION 56

Concerning cerebral ischaemia

A. Haemodilution can improve cerebral blood flow
B. Tirilizad mesylate can be used to reduce morbidity due to its glucocorticoid activity
C. The administration of nimodipine is of benefit to those with aneurysmal subarachnoid haemorrhage
D. N-methyl-D-aspartate (NMDA) antagonists have been shown to improve mortality
E. Cellular damage is mediated by low intracellular calcium concentrations

QUESTION 57

During the course of Guillain Barre syndrome (GBS)

A. The neuromuscular dysfunction is due to destruction of the neurone by a virus
B. Full recovery is the rule
C. Fisher's syndrome describes weakness without paraesthesia or sensory loss
D. Lumbar puncture is diagnostic
E. Plasmapheresis reduces the duration and severity of the acute phase

QUESTION 58

Chest tube drainage of the intrapleural space

A. Should be performed immediately if tension pneumothorax is suspected
B. Should be performed through the site of a penetrating chest injury
C. Producing a continued loss of 80 mls/hr of blood in an adult is an absolute indication for thoracotomy
D. Should pass immediately above a rib margin
E. Is indicated for the treatment of all pneumothoraces

QUESTION 59

Acute tubular necrosis (ATN) may follow

A. Burns
B. Falciparum malaria
C. Glucose-6-phosphate dehydrogenase deficiency
D. Diabetic ketoacidosis
E. Transfusion reaction

QUESTION 60

Concerning cardiogenic shock

- **A.** Defibrillation worsens overall prognosis
- **B.** The clinical findings occur when the cardiac index is less than 1.8 L/min/m²
- **C.** It can occur without the pulmonary capillary wedge pressure (PCWP) being elevated
- **D.** Intra-aortic counterpulsation with a balloon pump (IABP) is contra-indicated in patients with aortic stenosis
- **E.** When due to left ventricular infarction it is usually irreversible

QUESTION 61

Cellular uptake of potassium is stimulated by

- **A.** Acidosis
- **B.** Alpha-adrenergic stimulation
- **C.** Insulin
- **D.** Heparin
- **E.** Adrenaline

QUESTION 62

Concerning the care of patients with major trauma

- **A.** Over 80% of patients with spinal cord trauma develop deep vein thrombosis
- **B.** Early fracture fixation reduces the incidence of ARDS
- **C.** Glutamine is the preferred nutrient of the enterocyte and should be given to all enterally fed patients
- **D.** Up to 55% of patients staying 5 or more days will become colonized with potentially pathogenic micro-organisms
- **E.** If core temperature falls below 34 degrees centigrade the mortality is in the region of 40%

QUESTION 63

Pulmonary artery obstruction

- **A.** Following amniotic fluid embolism has a high mortality
- **B.** With air may require systemic anticoagulation following successful resuscitation
- **C.** Results in ST depression and T wave inversion in anterior leads on the ECG
- **D.** Is responsible for about 5% of all deaths
- **E.** May occur with choriocarcinoma

QUESTION 64

The following conditions can cause hyperlactatemia

A. Thiamine deficiency
B. Anaemia
C. Wilson's disease
D. Ethanol intoxication
E. Diabetes mellitus

QUESTION 65

Concerning disseminated intravascular coagulation (DIC)

A. It is characterized by the destruction of platelets in the spleen
B. It may present with thrombotic manifestations only
C. The definitive treatment is fresh frozen plasma
D. Cryoprecipitate contains concentrated factor V and fibrinogen
E. If heparin is used therapeutically the initial dose should be 50-100 units/kg

QUESTION 66

Sodium bicarbonate is indicated in the treatment of

A. Cardiac arrest
B. Drowning
C. Diabetic ketoacidosis
D. Uraemic acidosis
E. Renal tubular acidosis

QUESTION 67

The incidence of central venous catheter related bacteraemia

A. Can be reduced if a gown, cap and mask are used in addition to gloves and drapes
B. Is not affected by the type of site sterilising solution
C. Is reduced if the catheters are inserted and maintained by experienced staff
D. Is dramatically reduced if the dressing and infusate tubing are changed every day rather than every 3 days
E. Is no different if a catheter is changed over a guidewire every 3 days compared with fresh placement when clinically indicated

QUESTION 68

Concerning the management of a patient with an inhalational thermal injury

A. Arterial blood gases may be misleading
B. Airway obstruction may develop many hours after the initial injury
C. Steroids may be indicated
D. Early enteral feeding reduces the incidence of septic episodes
E. Selective decontamination of the digestive tract improves mortality rates

QUESTION 69

Nosocomial pneumonia

A. Is less common in Intensive Care Units than blood stream infections
B. Due to Pseudomonas aeriginosa is more common in those with chronic lung disease
C. Treatment in a patient with a history of influenza infection should include anti-staphylococcal agents
D. Can be diagnosed in an ICU patient with fever and purulent sputum
E. Is more likely to be caused by gram -ve pathogens if it occurs within 4 days of hospitalisation

QUESTION 70

During the course of a tetanus infection

A. If hypotension occurs, it is not due to the infection
B. GABAergic neurones are affected
C. Adequate sedation reduces the autonomic instability
D. A shorter incubation time is prognostically significant
E. Continuous nondepolarising neuromuscular blockade must be administered to the ventilated patient

QUESTION 71

Considering malignant hyperthermia during anaesthesia

A. Sevoflurane is a precipitant
B. The incidence is about 1 in 50,000 anaesthetics
C. Inheritance is by an autosomal dominant mechanism
D. Mannitol is added to vials of dantrolene to aid management of haemoglobinuria
E. Profound muscle weakness can result from the effect of dantrolene on calcium transport

QUESTION 72

Regarding CPR in adults

A. Lignocaine is routinely given intravenously in VF

B. The endotracheal tube dose of adrenaline is 2 - 3 mg

C. A massage to ventilation ratio of 5 : 2 is recommended

D. During asystole 5 mg of atropine should be given once only

E. During asystole 5 mg of adrenaline should be given if there is no response after 5 cycles

QUESTION 73

Considering the use of anaesthetic gas cylinders

A. There is no international colour code for gas cylinders

B. The filling ratio for nitrous oxide cylinders is less in temperate climates to avoid adverse pressure on the valve block

C. Cylinders are manufactured from aluminium for use in remote locations

D. The pin index sytem applies to cylinders up to size G

E. Carbon dioxide is stored as a liquid in equilibrium with its vapour

QUESTION 74

In the use of the circle system

A. An international standard dictates that a red coloured absorbant still has active CO_2 absorption capability

B. Fresh gas flow should be introduced downstream rather than upstream from the absorber

C. An 'in circle' vaporiser should be on the expiratory limb upstream of the absorber.

D. Resistance to gas flow in the system is dependent on respiratory rate

E. A fresh gas flow of >10 lpm is needed to denitrogenate the system prior to low flows

QUESTION 75

The Goldmann Cardiac Risk Index

A. Predicts risk of mortality following cardiac surgery

B. Includes a score for the presence of hypertension

C. Includes a score for the presence mitral valve disease

D. Includes a score for dysrhythmias

E. Includes a score for patient age

QUESTION 76

During anaesthesia for ECT

- **A.** Suxamethonium is given to decrease the seizure threshold
- **B.** A current of 30-45 J is used
- **C.** The preoperative use of monoamine oxidase inhibitors is a contraindication
- **D.** Following passage of the current there is intense parasympathetic activity
- **E.** Atropine should always be given prior to ECT

QUESTION 77

During carotid endarterectomy

- **A.** Surgery can be performed under regional anaesthesia, providing C2-C5 are blocked
- **B.** Halothane is the volatile agent of choice
- **C.** Opioids have no effect on cerebral blood flow
- **D.** EEG monitoring is an advantage
- **E.** Infiltration of the carotid body with lignocaine is helpful

QUESTION 78

In the electrocardiogram the QT interval

- **A.** Equals the length of atrial and ventricular contraction
- **B.** In its correction for heart rate is shortened by bradycardia
- **C.** Is shortened by digoxin therapy
- **D.** Is shortened in hyperkalaemia
- **E.** When lengthened is a risk factor for Torsade de Pointes

QUESTION 79

In patients undergoing transurethral resection of prostate

- **A.** Subarachnoid block up to T9 is required
- **B.** TURP is associated with a higher risk of death than open prostatectomy
- **C.** Regional anaesthesia confers a lower mortality then general anaesthesia
- **D.** GA is associated with a higher incidence of cognitive impairment than spinal anaesthesia
- **E.** Features of TUR syndrome include increased blood pressure and a slow pulse

QUESTION 80

During pregnancy

- **A.** Physiological anaemia is the result of fluid accumulation
- **B.** T wave inversion in leads V2 and V3 is normal
- **C.** The raised minute ventilation results from raised intra abdominal pressure
- **D.** There is an increased risk of hypoxaemia during anaesthesia
- **E.** Thromboembolic disease is the most common cause of death

QUESTION 81

In a patient with sickle cell anaemia

A. About 50% of their haemoglobin will be in the HbS form
B. Exchange transfusion is appropriate prior to major vascular surgery
C. Folate is contra-indicated perioperatively as it may provoke an aplastic crisis
D. The Hb-O_2 dissociation curve is shifted to the right aiding tissue O_2 unloading
E. The use of any tourniquet is absolutely contraindicated

QUESTION 82

During left sided single lung ventilation

A. Isoflurane causes a dose dependent decrease in hypoxic pulmonary vasoconstriction
B. All the pulmonary blood flow will go to the non dependent lung
C. There is an obligatory left to right shunt
D. Ketamine will impair arterial oxygenation
E. It is safe to allow a patient breathe spontaneously

QUESTION 83

Regarding analgesia during labour

A. Regional blockade of T10 – L2 is required during the first two stages
B. Paracervical block is associated with fetal arrhythmias
C. Nitrous oxide is useful in 80% of patients
D. The volume of the epidural space is reduced by the uterus
E. Intramuscular pethidine is safe within 4 hours of delivery

QUESTION 84

In anaesthesia for a patient with a mediastinal mass

A. A lymphoma is the most likely cause of superior vena cava compression
B. Dyspnoeic symptoms with superior vena cava compression indicate direct airway pressure
C. Direct compression of the cardiac chambers is common
D. Profound hypotension due to superior vena cava obstruction is the commonest complication
E. Airway compression is is most commonly due to lymphoma

QUESTION 85

During adult hypothermic cardiopulmonary bypass

A. Using temperature compensation for arterial blood gas analysis is called pH-stat analysis

B. CO_2 should be added to the oxygenator to maintain $PaCO_2$ at 40 mmHg measured at the patients temperature

C. Hypoglycaemia occurs due to increased insulin secretion

D. Aprotinin inhibits fibrinolysis by stimulation of plasmin

E. Haemodilution is lessened by using induced ventricular fibrillation to reduce myocardial damage

QUESTION 86

During posterior fossa surgery the risk of air embolus can be reduced by

A. Controlled hypotension

B. Fluid loading

C. Application of positive end expiratory pressure

D. Leg bandaging

E. The lateral as opposed to the prone position

QUESTION 87

When monitoring patients for intraoperative myocardial ischaemia

A. An oesophageal ECG lead is a sensitive method of detecting posterior wall ischaemia

B. A CM5 lead is most useful for monitoring anterior ischaemia

C. A CM5 lead requires the right arm electrode to be placed under the right clavicle

D. The standard three electrode system is designed to detect anterior ischaemia

E. Using a 5 electrode ECG only 50% of episodes of ischaemia will be detected

QUESTION 88

In the use of ventilators of the lungs

A. Pressure generators generate the high inspiratory pressures needed in patients with poor pulmonary compliance

B. Flow generators produce a constant inspiratory gas flow

C. Pressure and flow generators fall into exclusive groups

D. Using a 'jetting device' the driving gas is supplied at a pressure of 4 bar

E. The Manley ventilators are minute volume dividers

QUESTION 89

Assessing the severity of pain

A. The Magill Pain Questionnaire assesses the character of the pain but not the severity

B. Severity of pain is easily predictable from patient to patient

C. Visual Analogue Scores are not reliable in children under 10 years

D. Pain in neonates can be successfully assessed by measuring palmar sweating

E. Self-reporting of pain in children may be misleading

QUESTION 90

The Stellate Ganglion Block

A. Is a cervicothoracic sympathetic block

B. Provides vasodilatation of the ipsilateral arm

C. Is performed at the level of C4

D. Is likely to have been successful if the patients nasal breathing improves

E. Is performed medial to the carotid sheath

Exam 2: Answers

ANSWER   1

A. FALSE   B. FALSE   C. TRUE   D. TRUE   E. FALSE

Lactate dehydrogenase falls after about 10 days whereas aspartate transaminase falls after about 5 days. The female incidence is 1 per 1000, that of males is 3.5 per 1000. Hypotension is more likely to occur during a rapid infusion of streptokinase and responds by temporarily stopping the infusion and restarting it a slower rate. The temperature maybe raised up to 38.5 degress Celsius.

Ventricular arrythmias are the most common. 95% of patients have an arrythmia, 80% of which are ventricular ectopic beats.

Ref: Oh. Intensive Care Manual. 3rd edition. Butterworths. Part I.

ANSWER   2

A. TRUE   B. FALSE   C. TRUE   D. FALSE   E. TRUE

Surgical emphysema is air in the subcutaneous tissues which can be caused by pneumothorax or oesophageal rupture. The usual cause of spontaneous pneumothorax in patients over 40 years old is emphysema or COAD. It is due to rupture of lung bullae. Sudden onset of pleuritic chest pain with increasing breathlessness are the presenting features of pneumothorax. For large pneumothoraces (over 50% on chest X-ray) or a tension pneumothorax, a chest drain is indicated.

Ref: Hirsch, Yentis & Smith. Anaesthesia A to Z. Butterworth Heinemann. p 361
Kumar & Clark. Clinical Medicine. Balliere Tindall. Chapter 12

ANSWER   3

A. TRUE   B. FALSE   C. FALSE   D. TRUE   E. FALSE

Clinical jaundice is detectable over values of 50 micromol / l in caucasian skin, normal values being less than 17 micromol / l. Obstructive jaundice leads to pale stool due to the absence of bile pigments in the gut normally forming stercobilin. There is also dark urine due to a raised conjugated bilirubin spilling over into urine. Cirrhosis of the liver causes late jaundice, it is a poor prognostic sign. Carcinoma of the head of pancreas can cause an obstructive jaundice but contrary to older textbooks, pain is a feature and is felt in the back. Chlorpromazine causes jaundice due to intrahepatic cholestasis. It may occur several weeks after stopping the drug or even after a single dose.

Ref: Beck, Francis & Souhami. Tutorials in Differential Diagnosis. Churchill Livingstone. 2nd edition. p103

ANSWER   4

A. FALSE   B. TRUE   C. TRUE   D. TRUE   E. FALSE

Hyperthyroidism is associated with insomnia and nervousness. Hypercalcaemia occurs in 15% of cases of thyroid crisis, which is the life threatening clinical extreme of hyperthyroidism. Uncontrolled diabetes mellitus, infection, trauma, labour and eclampsia are provoking factors of hyperthyroidism. Pretibial myxoedema is a pink/brown subcutaneous infiltration of the lower leg found in hyperthyroidism. Tendon reflexes are brisk in hyperthyroidism.

Ref: Oh. Intensive Care Manual. 3rd edition. Butterworths. Part IV.
Yentis, Hirsh & Smith. Anaesthesia A to Z. Butterworth Heineman. p223.

ANSWER   5

A. FALSE   B. FALSE   C. TRUE   D. FALSE   E. FALSE

Hypercalcaemia causes cardiac arrythmias and a shortened QT interval. It also leads to constipation. Hypocalcaemia can cause a prolonged QT interval, positive Trousseau's sign and, if chronic, cataracts. Trousseau's sign is a characteristic posture where the fingers and thumb of the affected hand are held adducted and the hand is partially flexed at the metacarpophalangeal joints. The feet may be similarly affected. Ischaemia of the affected limb produced by a sphygmomanometer cuff inflated above the arterial pressure for 2 to 3 minutes will augment this sign or produce it if it is not already present.

Ref: Marshall. Clinical Chemistry. Lippincott Company. Ch 14

ANSWER   6

A. FALSE   B. TRUE   C. TRUE   D. FALSE   E. TRUE

Phaeochromocytomas are tumours of the sympathetic nervous system, 90% of which arise in the adrenal gland. Glycosuria is a feature of catecholamine excess. Signs and symptoms are frequently intermittent in nature. Vanillylmandelic acid (VMA) results from the enzymic breakdown of noradrenaline and adrenaline. Normal levels of VMA in three 24 hour urine collections virtually excludes the diagnosis of phaeochromocytoma.

Ref: Kumar & Clark. Clinical Medicine. Balliere Tindall. Ch16

ANSWER   7

A. FALSE   B. TRUE   C. TRUE   D. TRUE   E. TRUE

Carbon monoxide binds avidly to haemoglobin forming carboxyhaemoglobin (COHb) which gives a "cherry" red appearance. There is reduced oxygen transport which leads to tachycardia and angina as well as neurological symptoms and convulsions. Oxygen saturation on pulse oximetry is misleading as COHb is interpreted as oxygenated haemaglobin.

Ref: Yentis, Hirsch & Smith. Anaesthesia A to Z. Butterworth Heinemann. p73

ANSWER   8

A. TRUE   B. TRUE   C. FALSE   D. TRUE   E. FALSE

In chronic constrictive pericarditis a high filling pressure is essential to maintain cardiac output. This results in a raised venous pressure, tachycardia, peripheral oedema and ascites. It would be inappropriate to reduce this filling pressure. Primary treatment is surgical. Heart sounds are quiet and the apex is not usually palpable. Similar symptoms to malignant disease can occur, such as weight loss, hepatomegaly and ascites. The raised jugular venous pressure maybe mistaken for SVC obstruction.

Ref: Weatherall, Ledingham & Warrell. Oxford Textbook of Medicine. vol 2 section 13

ANSWER 9

A. FALSE   B. TRUE   C. TRUE   D. TRUE   E. TRUE

Air in the pleural cavity increases resonance in proportion to the amount present. Pleural effusions cause a characteristic "stony" dullness over the effusion. Pulmonary TB may lead to diminshed resonance over the affected apex due to local infiltration and fibrosis. Infection causing consolidation diminishes resonance as the underlying lung is more solid. Oedema due to heart failure is usually basal and may be dull to percussion.

Ref: Swash & Mason. Hutchinson's Clinical Methods. 18th edition. Balliere Tindall Ch 8

ANSWER 10

A. TRUE   B. FALSE   C. FALSE   D. FALSE   E. TRUE

These indices indicate a microcytic anaemia (normal MCV = 85 fl). The most common cause is iron deficiency. The red cells will also be hypochromic (MCH less than 27 pg). In thalassaemia there is a deficiency in the synthesis of the globin chains of haemoglobin. In addition the accumulation of abnormal chains within the red cell leads to its early destruction. This causes an anaemia with reduced MCV and MCH. The reticulocyte count is also raised. The anaemia of renal failure is normocytic and normochromic, in common with anaemias of chronic disease. In renal failure it is due to reduced erythropoietin production and in severe uraemia, >30 mmol/l, a shortened red cell life and marrow toxicity. Folate and vitamin B12 deficiency cause macrocytic (high MCV) megaloblastic anaemia. Acute blood loss will cause an anaemia with a normal MCV and normal shaped existing red cells

Ref: Kumar, Clarke. Clinical Medicine. Balliere Tindall.

ANSWER 11

A. TRUE   B. TRUE   C. TRUE   D. FALSE   E. TRUE

During insufflation with carbon dioxide a 30% increase in arterial tension may occur. Minute ventilation may need to be increased to prevent hypercarbia. Insufflation of air during closure of the abdomen can cause sub-diaphragmatic nitrogen accumulation (since it is insoluble) which can take a long time to be resorbed and can cause referred shoulder-tip pain. The use of the Trendelenburg position is associated with a 20% fall in FRC. Peritoneal stimulation may cause bradycardia or asystole. Diaphragmatic splinting and impaired venous return occur with pneumoperitoneum. Venous return is initially enhanced by head down position and mild intrabdominal pressure rise but may be diminished by excessive insufflation pressure.

Ref: Craft & Upton. Key Topics in Anaesthesia. Bios Scientific Publications.

ANSWER   12

A. TRUE   B. TRUE   C. FALSE   D. TRUE   E. TRUE

Patients with obstructive jaundice have a high operative morbidity and mortality. Post-operative mortality is increased if the patient has malignant disease, if the plasma bilirubin >200 umol/l, and if the haematocrit < 30%. Raised alkaline phosphatase suggests extra-hepatic obstruction whereas raised transaminases suggest hepatocellular damage. Biliary obstruction causes reduced vitamin K absorption and hence coagulopathy secondary to reduced synthesis of clotting factors II, VII, IX and X. Thus, extra-dural anaesthesia is contraindicated.

Ref: McLatchie. Oxford Handbook of Clinical Surgery. Oxford University Press.

ANSWER   13

A. TRUE   B. FALSE   C. TRUE   D. FALSE   E. TRUE

The risk of DVT increases linearly with age in patients over 40 undergoing major surgery. Virchow (1856) described a triad of risk factors: venous stasis, vessel wall damage, and increased coagulability. Myeloma causes increased blood viscosity and therefore venous stasis. Other causes of venous stasis include prolonged immobility (eg paraplegia), pelvic venous obstruction, low cardiac output. Causes of vessel wall damage include direct trauma and inflammation. There are many causes of increased blood coagulability, including trauma, malignancy, puerperium, oestrogen administration and hereditary hypercoagulability (eg Protein C deficiency). The mini-pill is progesterone only and therefore does not present a major risk factor.

Ref: Yentis Hirsch and Smith. Anaesthesia A to Z. Butterworth Heinemann.

ANSWER   14

A. TRUE   B. TRUE   C. FALSE   D. FALSE   E. FALSE

Findings that suggest a cervical cord injury include flaccid areflexia, diaphragmatic breathing, ability to flex but not extend at the elbow, hypotension, bradycardia and priapism. Neurogenic shock results from impairment of the descending sympathetic pathway in the spinal cord resulting in loss of vasomotor tone and sympathetic innervation to the heart. This results in hypotension and bradycardia in the absence of hypovolaemia. Treatment with vasopressors is advocated. The corticospinal tract is in the posterolateral aspect of the cord and controls ipsilateral motor power. Spinal shock occurs shortly after spinal injury even if the cord is not completely destroyed. Initial flaccidity and areflexia gives way to spasticity after days or weeks.

Most thoracic vertebral fractures from T1 to T10 are stable because of the rigidity of the rib cage. From T11 to L1 most are unstable.

Ref. Advanced Trauma Life Support Student Manual. American College of Surgeons.

ANSWER   15

A. FALSE   B. TRUE   C. TRUE   D. FALSE   E. FALSE

Tracheo-oesophageal fistula has an incidence of 1 in 3500 births with an equal sex incidence. The commonest type (85%) involve oesophageal atresia. It is diagnosed by passing a radio-opaque nasogastric tube into the blind pouch. Contrast medium is avoided because of the risk of aspiration. A right thoracotomy with an extra-pleural approach is used during surgical correction. Tracheomalacia is a complication after repair.

Ref: Yentis Hirsch and Smith. Anaesthesia A to Z. Butterworth Heinemann.

ANSWER 16

A. TRUE   B. TRUE   C. TRUE   D. TRUE   E. TRUE

Both ulcerative colitis and crohns disease carry an increased risk of developing carcinoma of the large bowel, the risks with ulcerative colitis being greater. Familial polyposis coli is an autosomal dominant condition in which malignant change is inevitable, although unknown before the age of 20 years. Total colectomy is performed. Plummer-Vinson syndrome consists of iron-deficiency anaemia and dysphagia due to the presence of an oesophageal web. It predisposes to oesophageal carcinoma. Adenomatous villi account for 10% of neoplastic polyps of the large bowel.

Ref: Forrest, Carter and McLeod. Principles and Practise of Surgery. Churchill Livingstone.

ANSWER 17

A. FALSE   B. TRUE   C. FALSE   D. TRUE   E. TRUE

Coronary artery bypass grafting is performed for ischaemic heart disease unresponsive to medical therapy. Both saphenous vein grafts (reversed because of valves) and internal mammary artery grafts are used, often in combination. IMA grafts provide prolonged patency but are associated with more post-operative bleeding. Life expectancy post CABG is improved in stenosis of the left mainstem coronary artery, double vessel disease involving severe proximal stenosis of the left anterior descending coronary artery, triple vessel disease, moderate/severe angina and impaired left ventricular function. Life expectancy is not improved where angina is not present pre-operatively. The mortality of CABG is < 1% for two grafts in a patient with no intercurrent disease. It rises with increasing number of grafts, previous infarctions and impaired LV function as well as with intercurrent disease. The mortality of CABG is higher in women.

Ref: Yentis Hirsch and Smith. Anaesthesia A to Z. Butterworth Heinemann.

ANSWER 18

A. TRUE   B. TRUE   C. FALSE   D. TRUE   E. TRUE

Acute appendicitis is the commonest abdominal emergency in the UK affecting 1/6th of the population. Nothing can be so easy, nor anything so difficult as the diagnosis! It usually presents with constipation, but diarrhoea can occur. Referred pain from a basal pneumonia can mimic acute appendicitis. It usually causes a leucocytosis with a neutrophilia but the white cell count can be normal. Microscopic haematuria occurs if the inflamed appendix is adherent to the bladder or ureter.

Ref: Ellis and Calne. Lecture notes on General Surgery. Blackwell Scientific Publications.

ANSWER 19

A. TRUE   B. TRUE   C. TRUE   D. FALSE   E. FALSE

Methylmethacrylate is the acrylic cement used in orthopaedic surgery. The cause of hypotension, hypoxaemia or cardiovascular collapse on its application is unknown. Possible explanations include allergic reaction, peripheral vasodilatation, fat or air embolism due to high pressures generated in the bone cavity or direct cardio-toxicity of the monomer. Risks are reduced by fluid preloading prior to insertion, using a cement gun to apply the cement hence avoiding air trapping in the bone cavity and washing out the cavity with saline prior to insertion.

Ref: Yentis Hirsch and Smith. Anaesthesia A toZ. Butterworth Heinemann.

ANSWER 20

A. FALSE   B. FALSE   C. FALSE   D. FALSE   E. TRUE

Breast, lung and testicular primaries commonly metastasise to brain.

Ref: McLatchie. Oxford Handbook of Clinical Surgery. Oxford University Press.

ANSWER 21

A. TRUE   B. TRUE   C. FALSE   D. FALSE   E. TRUE

Midazolam is only available in the injectable form in the UK although it is effective orally. A dose of 0.07-0.08 mg/kg intramuscularly produces sedation and anxiolysis. Cyclizine, in common with domperidone and metoclopramide, increases lower oesophageal sphincter tone. Awareness during Caesarean section is less common when hyoscine is administered compared with atropine. Rectal thiopentone has been used to sedate children, but it is unpredictable, so the patient should be supervised between administration and handover to the anaesthetist. Atropine antagonises both the hastened gastric motility and the increase in lower oesophageal sphincter tone usually produced by metoclopramide.

Ref: Vickers, Morgan and Spencer. Drugs in Anaesthetic Practice (Seventh Edition) Butterworth-Heinemann Ltd. Ch 2 and 3.

ANSWER 22

A. TRUE   B. FALSE   C. FALSE   D. TRUE   E. TRUE

Genetic variations of plasma cholinesterase are due to the atypical, fluoride, silent and other genes. The heterozygous state for the atypical gene is present in 4% of the Caucasian population and is the most common variant. The hetrozygous state for the fluoride gene is present in 0.5%. Both cause only slight prolongation of the action of suxamethonium.

Dibucaine inhibits the normal action of plasma cholinesterase on benzoylcholine, the percentage inhibition is known as the dibucaine number. Therefore, patients with the normal homzygous structure of plasma cholinesterase have a high dibucaine number- above 77. Patients heterozygous for the atypical gene have a dibucaine number of 54-70.

Although an anticholinesterase may reduce the length of neuromuscular blockade if features of a non-depolarising block are present, it is generally recommended that this is not given as it may further complicate the situation. Approximately 17% of prolonged apnoeas following suxamethonium may be due to acquired decreases in plasma cholinesterase activity. This may be due to pregnancy, renal and liver disorders, hypothyroidism and drugs that are also metabolised by plasma cholinesterase e.g. neostigmine, etomidate, ester local anaesthetic agents and methotrexate.

Ref: Nimmo, Rowbotham and Smith. Anaesthesia (Second Edition) Blackwell Scientific Publications. Ch 14.

ANSWER 23

A. FALSE   B. FALSE   C. FALSE   D. TRUE   E. FALSE

Mivacurium consists of three stereoisomers, trans-trans, cis-trans and cis-cis. Clearance of the cis-trans and trans-trans isomers correlate strongly with plasma cholinesterase activity but the cis-cis isomer has a low plasma clearance.Mivacurium's duration of action varies inversely with plasma cholinesterase activity and in patients with cirrhosis plasma clearances of the cis-trans and trans-trans isomers are decreased but that of the cis-cis isomer is unchanged. Mivacurium has been used in myasthenic patients but with lower initial and maintanence doses. Atracurium consists of ten isomers.

Ref: Current Opinion in Anaesthesiology 1995:Vol 8, No4

ANSWER 24

A. FALSE   B. FALSE   C. TRUE   D. TRUE   E. FALSE

Drugs delivered by the transdermal route must have lipid solubility to pass through the stratum corneum (outermost, lipophilic layer of skin) and aqueous solubility to pass through the dermis.

Oral and nasal transmucosal drug delivery requires drugs that are lipophlic, unionised and of small molecular weight. There is rapid absorption and no first-pass metabolism. Fentanyl is rapidly absorbed through the nasal mucosa with onset of analgesia within ten minutes. The analgesia is nearly as effective as the same dose of intravenous fentanyl. Midazolam is only licensed for parenteral administration. However, it is effective orally (swallowed) in a dose of 0.5-0.75 mg/kg but is very bitter to taste and needs to be diluted with, for example, concentrated blackcurrant juice. Intranasal administration requires a dose of 0.1-0.3 mg/kg but again is limited by the bitter taste most patients experience and a burning sensation. Transdermal scopolamine is administered for motion sickness and has been used for postoperative nausea and vomiting. Effective drug concentrations are not achieved for 6-8 hours. Post-auricular skin is 20 times more permeable to scopolamine than the thigh, and therefore patients are instructed to place the patch behind their ear.

Ref: Streisand JB, Stanley TH. Newer drug delivery systems. Current Anaesthesia and Critical Care 1995;6:113-120

ANSWER 25

A. TRUE   B. FALSE   C. TRUE   D. TRUE   E. FALSE

Antipsychotic drugs vary in their tendency to cause side effects. Chlorpromazine is associated with a high incidence of sedation and hypotension, haloperidol and pimozide with movement disorders, whereas risperidone tends to cause fewer problems and has no anticholinergic effects. Movement disorders are due to D_2 receptor blockade, and manifest as akathisia (restlessness), dystonias (increase in muscle tone), pseudo-parkinsonism and tardive dyskinesia (choreo-athetoid mouth movements). Dystonias and pseudo-parkinsonism can be treated with anticholinergic drugs including procyclidine, benztropine or orphenadrine.

Ref: Livingston MG. Management of schizophrenia. Prescribers' Journal 1996;36:206-215

ANSWER 26

A. FALSE   B. TRUE   C. TRUE   D. TRUE   E. FALSE

Benzodiazepines are almost entirely eliminated from the body by hepatic metabolism. This usually involves oxidative reactions but some, for example oxazepam, are almost entirely eliminated by glucuronide conjugation. The following have active metabolites

Flunitrazepam, Flurazepam, Loprazolam, Triazolam, Alprazolam, Bromazepam, Chlordiazepoxide, Clobazam, Diazepam, Ketazolam, Medazepam and Prazepam. Minor amounts of temazepam (2%) may be metabolized to oxazepam.

Ref: Calvey and Wiliams. Principles and Practice of Pharmacology for Anaesthetists. Blackwell Scientific Publications. Ch12

ANSWER   27
A. FALSE   B. TRUE   C. FALSE   D. TRUE   E. FALSE

Bretylium may be used as a second line agent for the treatment of ventricular dysrhythmias resistant to lignocaine. Its side effects include hypotension, nausea and vomiting. Paraquat causes local effects such as mucosal and skin irritation and systemic effects including vomiting, diarrhoea, renal failure and pulmonary fibrosis. Corticosteroids may be beneficial in the treatment of pulmonary fibrosis. A major disadvantage of bleomycin is the dose related emergence of progressive pulmonary fibrosis. High inspired oxygen concentrations during general anaesthesia may lead to respiratory failure. Chloroquine may cause GI disturbances, headache, convulsions, visual disturbances, skin rashes, bone-marrow suppression, retinal damage, corneal opacities and ECG changes.

Ref: British National Formulary. 1996;32

ANSWER   28
A. FALSE   B. FALSE   C. FALSE   D. FALSE   E. FALSE

Nitric oxide is synthesised from L-arginine in an enzymatically controlled process by nitric oxide synthase which has a variety of forms. Changes in flow do lead to production of nitric oxide although basal tone is suggested to be little influenced by nitric oxide in the coronary circulation. It does not directly affect Ca^{++} channels but does so by a production of cGMP by the activation of guanylate cyclase. It has a half life of seconds since it has a high affinity for haemoglobin with the formation of methaemoglobin, a process which leads to its inactivation.

Ref: Prys-Roberts & Brown. International Practice of Anaesthesia. Chapter 22. The heart - Myocardial metabolism and contraction - ventricular function.

ANSWER   29
A. FALSE   B. FALSE   C. TRUE   D. FALSE   E. TRUE

The pressure difference from mouth to pleural cavity during spontaneous breathing is produced by lowering pleural pressure. Therefore, during IPPV, mean intrathoracic pressure must be higher. Right ventricular filling falls during IPPV, the effect of this on cardiac output depends upon the blood volume and the integrity of the sympathetic nervous system to control peripheral vasculature. PEEP may maintain alveolar patency, lung inflation may open collapsed airways. During IPPV there is a transmural pressure difference between the intra and extra thoracic aorta. This results in a reduced afterload improving patients in left ventricular failure.

Ref: Scurr, Feldman and Soni. Scientific Foundations of Anaesthesia 4th ed. Heinemann. Ch 25 pp 297.

ANSWER   30
A. FALSE   B. FALSE   C. TRUE   D. TRUE   E. FALSE

Atropine blocks the action of the vagus and has an antisialogogue effect. Cimetidine is an H_2 receptor blocker and reduces gastric acidity. Antacids neutralise secreted acid but may have to be given regularly to increase pH above 5. Osmotic particles in radiopaque dyes or bowel preparations increase losses of fluids via the gut and can lead to profound dehydration in the elderly. Diuretics have no direct actions on gastrointestinal secretions.

Ref: Harrison,Healy and Thornton. Aids to Anaesthesia. Churchill Livingstone. pp186

ANSWER 31

A. TRUE   B. FALSE   C. TRUE   D. FALSE   E. FALSE

Haemoglobin from disrupted red blood cells is phagocytosed by macrophages. It is then split into globin and haem. The latter is split into iron and a chain of pyrrole nuclei from which biliverdin is formed. Bilirubin is derived and released into the plasma where it immediately combines with albumin and is transported to the liver. In the hepatocyte 80% of bilirubin is conjugated with glucuronic acid and 10% with sulphate. Bilirubin is then released conjugated into cannaliculi and passes to the intestine. 50% of conjugated bilirubin is converted to urobilinogen some of which is reabsorbed into the blood. 5% is renally excreted with the remainder being re-excreted by the liver. In obstructive jaundice conjugated bilirubin will be released into the blood and will appear in the urine where it can be detected by foaming the urine, the foam then being yellow.

Ref: Guyton and Hall. Textbook of Medical Physiology. Chapter 70. The liver as an organ.

ANSWER 32

A. FALSE   B. FALSE   C. FALSE   D. TRUE   E . TRUE

During apnoea the $PaCO_2$ rises by 3 - 6 mmHg per minute (0.5-0.8 kPa). It is produced by aerobic respiration at a rate determined at rest by the basal metabolic rate. During apnoea, failure of ventilation leads to an equilibration of mixed venous, alveolar and arterial PCO_2. Alveolar oxygen will be progressively consumed at approximately 250 ml / min.

Ref: Nunn. Applied Respiratory Physiology. Butterworths

ANSWER 33

A. FALSE   B.FALSE   C. TRUE   D. TRUE   E. TRUE

Diastole is divided into active relaxation, rapid filling, slow filling and atrial systole. Active relaxation is improved by sympathetic stimulation, increased inotropic state and increased heart rate. In the early part of diastole 70% of ventricular filling occurs. Especially when the left ventricle is hypertrophied any increase in heart rate will adversely affect left ventricular filling. Ventricular filling is most commonly disturbed by hypertensive heart disease and myocardial infarction. A modulus of chamber stiffness is the slope of the (dp/dv)/P relationship for the exponential curve of diastolic pressure against volume.

Ref: Priebe & Skarvan. Cardiovascular Physiology. BMJ Publishing. Chapter 2. Ventricular performance.

ANSWER 34

A. FALSE   B. TRUE   C. TRUE   D. TRUE   E. TRUE

Hepatic blood flow is normally 500 ml/min from the hepatic artery and 1300ml/min via the portal system. Splanchnic autoregulation is not as prononunced as in some specialised circulations, however decreased blood flow is ameliorated by a form of post ischaemic hyperperfusion. A variety of circulating substances also dilate the splanchnic circulation including most of the gastro-intestinal peptides. Vasoconstriction of the splanchnic circulation induced by catecholamines only occurs during times of shock. Renal autoregulation is either achieved by myogenic control or tubuloglomerular feedback involving tubular Na^+ delivery and renin release. PgE_2 and PgI_2 are locally produced during haemorrhagic hypovolaemia and vasodilating afferent and efferent arterioles so reducing ischaemia.

Ref: Priebe and Skarvan. Cardiovascular Physiology. Renal, Splanchnic, skin and muscle circulations.

ANSWER 35

A. TRUE   B. FALSE   C. TRUE   D. FALSE   E. FALSE

Acidosis is a condition in which the hydrogen ion concentration is raised, acidaemia is a lower than normal plasma pH. Metabolic acidosis is caused by increased hydrogen ion production or ingestion, failure to excrete hydrogen ions, or loss of bicarbonate. Compensation is by hyperventilation and increased renal excretion. Treatment is of the underlying cause. Bicarbonate therapy is sometimes useful, but controversial.

Ref: Yentis, Hirsch, Smith. Anaesthesia A-Z. Butterworth. pp4.

ANSWER 36

A. FALSE   B. FALSE   C. TRUE   D. TRUE   E. FALSE

The arterioles are the site of greatest vascular resistance within the kidney, but this is lower than in other organs. As a consequence there is always blood flow in all renal capillaries. The cells responsible for the secretion of renin are within the media of the afferent arteriole. Renin is secreted in response to a fall in renal perfusion pressure, a rise in tubular sodium concentration and sympathetic nervous stimulation. Renin secretion will result in the production of angiotensin II (50 times more potent as a vasoconstrictor than noradrenaline with a half life of 30 secs). It causes a fall in renal blood flow and sodium retention as a result of aldosterone secretion. GFR is dependent on blood flow and is controlled by the balance of the afferent and efferent arterioles. Oncotic pressure rises along the length of the glomerular capillary decreasing filtration. Capillary permeabilty is about 10 -100 higher in the glomerulus.

Ref: Scurr. Feldman, and Soni. Scientific Foundations 4th ed. Heineman. pp 410-412

ANSWER 37

A. TRUE   B. TRUE   C. TRUE   D. TRUE   E. TRUE

The extradural space extends from the foramen magnum to the sacrococcygeal membrane of the sacral canal. It contains extradural fat, extradural veins (Batson's plexus), lymphatics and spinal nerve roots. Connective tissue layers have been demonstrated within the extradural space sometimes dividing it into right and left portions.

Ref. Yentis Hirsch and Smith. Anaesthesia A to Z.Butterworth Heinemann. p173

ANSWER 38

A. TRUE   B. FALSE   C. FALSE   D. FALSE   E. TRUE

The intercostal spaces are served by anterior intercostal arteries (from the internal thoracic artery) and the posterior intercostal arteries (the lower 9 from the aorta and the upper 2 from the superior intercostal artery). The intercostal nerves are the primary anterior rami of the thoracic spinal nerves. They are mixed, motor (to the intercostal muscle) and sensory (serving skin). From above downwards in the costal groove lie the intercostal vein, artery and nerve. These lie between the internal intercostal muscles and the transverse thoracis muscle.

Ref. Snell. Clinical Anatomy For Medical Students. Little Brown. Boston.

ANSWER 39

A. FALSE   B. FALSE   C. TRUE   D. TRUE   E. FALSE

The stellate ganglion represents the fused inferior cervical and first thoracic sympathetic ganglia. It is present in 80% of subjects. Stellate ganglion block is performed for painful conditions of the arm e.g. reflex sympathetic dystrophy and phantom limb pain as well as to improve circulation in the arm in conditions such as Raynaud's disease and post embolectomy. It may also help to relieve the pain of herpes zoster infections of the head and neck and has been advocated as a means of reducing post thoracotomy pain by blocking sympathetic sensory fibres to the pleural cavity. It lies on the flat lateral border of the vertebral body of C7. When preparing to block it, the patient is placed in the supine position and the transverse process of the 6th cervical vertebra (Chassaignac's tubercle) palpated. This lies approximately 2cm lateral to the cricoid cartilage. The carotid sheath is retracted laterally and the needle inserted posteriorly to contact bone. It is withdrawn 1-2mm and the local anaesthetic solution injected. Success is denoted by the onset of Horner's syndrome. Complications include intravascular injection, recurrent laryngeal and brachial plexus blocks, pneumothorax, subarachnoid and extradural injection, and haematoma formation.

Ref. Yentis, Hirsch and Smith. Anaesthesia A to Z. Butterworth Heinemann.

ANSWER 40

A. TRUE   B. FALSE   C. TRUE   D. FALSE   E. TRUE

The first rib is one of the shortest and most curved of all ribs. It has a superior surface marked by two shallow depressions separated by a rough surface for the attachment of scalenus anterior. The anterior depression transmits the subclavian vein and the posterior depression the subclavian artery. The first rib is a true rib because it is connected behind with the vertebral column and in front with the sternum via the costal cartilages. It has no angle but at this place the rib is slightly bent with the convexity of the bend upwards, so the head of the bone is directed downwards. The under surface is smooth and has no grooves.

Ref. Pick and Howden. Gray's Anatomy. Galley Press.

ANSWER 41

A. FALSE   B. TRUE   C. TRUE   D. TRUE   E. TRUE

The exercise or stress ECG is useful if the normal 12 lead ECG demonstrates no abnormality and the patient is known to develop symptoms on exercise. The exercise load is started at an easily managed level and then is incrementally increased in 1.5-3 minute stages with the aim of exhausting the subject within 15 minutes. BP and ECG are monitored continuously. The test is conclusively positive if angina is accompanied by >2mm downsloping ST segment depression. A drop in BP is diagnostic of severe ischaemia. Sensitivity is 30% with simple step tests but 75-96% with cycle or treadmill protocols. Specificity is low in asymptomatic patients but higher in men with angina. A false positive rate of 10-25% has been demonstrated in healthy women.

Ref: Kaufman L. Anaesthesia Review 10. (Churchill Livingstone) Ch1.

ANSWER 42

A. FALSE   B. FALSE   C. FALSE   D. TRUE   E. TRUE

Direct measurement allows beat-by-beat assessment of arterial pressure. A continuous flush device is used that delivers 2-3ml/hr through the cannula. Damping within the measurement system should be optimal, rather than critical as the latter does not allow a fast enough response to see a normal waveform and an accurate systolic pressure. Accurate reproduction of amplitude is easy for the mean but more difficult for systolic and diastolics. Systems in clinical use, commonly have a natural frequency of 15Hz. When undamped, sine waves are reproduced accurately up to driving frequencies of only about 20% of the natural frequency (ie 3Hz). Optimal damping allows reproduction of sine waves to within to 2% of their original AMPLITUDE at driving frequencies of up to 10Hz (ie 2/3 of the natural frequency of the system). When heart rate rises or examination of the SHAPE of the waveform is critical, optimally damped systems with natural frequencies of up to 60Hz may be required.

Ref: Parbrook, G.D. and Gray, W.M. (1990) The Measurement of Blood Pressure. In: Scurr, C., Feldman, S. and Soni, N. (Eds.) Scientific Foundations of Anaesthesia; The Basis of Intensive Care, 4th edn. pp. 70-81. Oxford: Heinemann Medical Books. Nimmo & Smith. Anaesthesia. Ch27. (Blackwell).

ANSWER 43

A. TRUE   B. TRUE   C. FALSE   D. FALSE   E. FALSE

Blood gas analysers now commonly incorporate a pH, oxygen and carbon dioxide electrode. All are maintained at 37 degrees centigrade by a thermal control system. Dissociation of acids and bases increase with temperature so may give false results. A correction factor maybe used to indicate the true hydrogen ion concentration in a hypothermic patient. Both the hydrogen ion and carbon dioxide measurement systems consist of a glass electrode sensitive to hydrogen ions. The hydrogen ion system consists of a silver / silver chloride electrode in contact with a solution of chloride ions whereas the carbon dioxide electrode consists of the glass in contact with a bicarbonate buffer. The measurement of carbon dioxide is dependent on the dissociation of carbon dioxide into hydrogen ions. Hence the response time of this electrode is greater than the hydrogen ion electrode alone. The oxygen electrode (Clarke or polargraphic electrode) consists of a platinum cathode and a silver / silver chloride anode in a solution such as potassium chloride. A plastic membrane separates blood from the cathode hence preventing protein deposits forming on it.

Ref: Davis, Parbrook, Kenny. Basic Physics and Measurement in Anaesthesia. 4th Edition. Butterworth Heinemann.

ANSWER 44

A. FALSE   B. TRUE   C. TRUE   D. TRUE   E. FALSE

Haemoglobinopathies that have been investigated (HbF, HbS and HbH) appear to have no effect on pulse oximetry. Blue or green dyes including methylene blue cause a transient fall in SpO_2. Haemoglobin levels below 14.5 g/dl cause a progressive under estimation of SaO_2. As oximeters cannot be calibrated in humans at low oxygen saturations there is progressive inaccuracy below 60%, with most machines under-reading. Jaundice does not affect SpO_2.

Ref: Moon, R.E. and Camporesi, E.M. (1990) Respiratory Monitoring. In: Miller, R.D. (Ed.) Anesthesia, 3rd edn. pp. 1129-1163. New York: Churchill Livingstone

ANSWER 45

A. TRUE   B. FALSE   C. TRUE   D. FALSE   E. TRUE

Infra-red absorption eg by carbon dioxide, nitrous oxide and the volatiles is used in capnography. The amount of light absorbed is measured indirectly by comparison with reference gas or by detection of sound emitted by excited molecules (photoacoustic spectroscopy). With an interferometer a light beam is split and passed through 2 chambers, one reference and the other sample. The beams are delayed to different extents, thus the emergent beams are out of phase. The resultant interference pattern is visualised through a telescope, and is displaced when gas is drawn into the sample chamber. Degree of change is related to the sample concentration. Concentration of vapours can be measured by adsorption onto rubber strips eg Drager Narkotest. Chromatography can be used to measure carbon dioxide levels. It uses the principle of separation of the sample's component gases depending upon its solubility in 2 phases ie an inert carrier gas and a column of silica alumina particles coated in oil or wax. The polargraphic cell is used to measure oxygen.

Ref: Yentis, Hirsch, Smith. Anaesthesia A to Z. Butterworth Heinemann.

ANSWER 46

A. TRUE   B. FALSE   C. FALSE   D. TRUE   E. TRUE

The distal lumen of a pulmonary artery catheter has a maximum natural frequency of 12 Hz, causing significant errors due to resonance at high heart rates.

LVSW is stroke volume (SV) x mean systolic pressure (MAP) x 0.0144.

SVRI is 79.92 x (MAP - CVP) / Cardiac Index

which is also 79.92 x (MAP - CVP) x (BSA / Cardiac Output)

The derived PVR is a poor indicator of the resistance to pulsatile flow. Furthermore it relies on pressure values that have a large degree of error. Sepsis classically causes vasodilation (and a low SVR).

Ref: Runciman, W.B. (1989) Monitoring. In: Nimmo, W.S. and Smith, G. (Eds.) Anaesthesia, pp. 460-491. Oxford: Blackwell Scientific Publications

ANSWER 47

A. TRUE   B. TRUE   C. TRUE   D. TRUE   E. TRUE

Low amplitude temperature / time curves result when the injectate volume is too small (less than 10 ml) or the temperature differential between injectate and patient is small. This may occur if the injectate is inadvertently warmed in a syringe placed in the palm during injection.

Tricuspid or pulmonary regurgitation and intracardiac shunts may produce recirculation errors. A diminished height of the concentration/time curve can occur from incomplete filling of the syringe, loss of injectate through leaks or a thrombus insulating the pulmonary artery thermistor. Each of these results in a falsely high cardiac output reading.

Ref: Barash, Cullen, Stoelting. Clinical Anesthesia. 2nd Edition. J.B. Lippincott Company.

ANSWER 48

A. FALSE   **B. FALSE**   **C. FALSE**   **D. FALSE**   **E. TRUE**

Tetanic fade, a progressive reduction in the height of twitches in a train-of-four, and post-tetanic potentiation are all features of non-depolarising blockade. Pancuronium, like other non-depolarising blocking agents antagonises depolarising block, whereas anticholinesterases potentiate the block. Progression of depolarising block to a state that has the features of non-depolarising block is called dual or phase II block.

Ref: Hudes, E. and Lee, K.C. (1987) Clinical use of peripheral nerve stimulators in anaesthesia. Canadian Journal of Anaesthesia 34, 525-534.

ANSWER 49

A. TRUE   **B. FALSE**   **C. FALSE**   **D. FALSE**   **E. TRUE**

ACT can be measured in theatre using an automated system such as the Haemochron. 2ml of blood is mixed with 12mg of diatomaceous earth (a fine powder providing a large surface area for conversion of factor XII to XIIa). The end point occurs normally after 70-110 seconds when a clot is formed that prevents a magnetic rod in the bottle from maintaining the contacts between a switch in the base of the machine. The unit must be heated to 37C to maintain reliable results. Hypothermic samples should be warmed or a correction applied. Haemodilution will also prolong the ACT. Although inter-patient response to heparin varies, individual dose responses are linear. An ACT of >400 seconds is required to prevent coagulation in an oxygen reservoir filter.

Ref:Miller RD. Anesthesia (Churchill Livingstone) Ch31.

ANSWER 50

A. TRUE   **B. TRUE**   **C. FALSE**   **D. TRUE**   **E. TRUE**

The EEG is caused by potentials mainly generated in the pyramidal cells at a depth of about 800 Åm. The awake EEG is predominantly alpha in 75-90% of individuals. The EEG is affected by intracerebral structural lesions, trauma, cerebrovascular disease, hypoxia, hypercarbia, hypoglycemia as well as many drugs. These include all anaesthetic induction and inhalational agents as well as all opioids. The changes seen with enflurane are described in the question.

Ref: Hoffman, W.E. and Grundy, B.L. (1990) Physiology of the Electroencephalogram. In: Scurr, C., Feldman, S. and Soni, N. (Eds.) Scientific Foundations of Anaesthesia; The Basis of Intensive Care, 4th edn. pp. 325-345. Oxford: Heinemann Medical Books

ANSWER 51

A. TRUE   **B. TRUE**   **C. FALSE**   **D. TRUE**   **E. FALSE**

Sepsis, infection, bacteraemia, septic shock and the systemic inflammatory response syndrome (SIRS) are often terms used interchangeably. There are calls, however, to agree on stricter terminology. Infection = inflammatory response against microorganisms or invasion of sterile host tissue by these organisms. Bacteraemia = viable bacteria in the blood. SIRS = a response to a number of insults. Sepsis = systemic response to infection. Both the latter two include at least two of the following: temperature disturbance, tachycardia, tachypnoea and white cell count abnormalities. Severe sepsis = sepsis associated with organ dysfunction, hypoperfusion or hypotension. Septic shock = sepsis with hypotension and hypoperfusion despite adequate fluid resuscitation. In septicaemia multiple organs may be affected. There may be depression in conscious level, fever or hypothermia, hypotension (despite an initial rise in the cardiac index), supraventricular dysrhythmias (in 40%), tachypnoea, hypoxia, oliguria, jaundice, stress ulceration and thrombocytopaenia. Current evidence points to an increase in the production of the free radical nitric oxide, causing vascular relaxation via cyclic guanosine monophosphate.

Ref: Hillman and Bishop. Clinical Intensive Care. Cambridge University Press. Ch 13. American College of Chest Physicians/Society of Critical Care Medicine Consensus Conference: Definitions for sepsis and organ failure and guidelines for the use of innovative therapies in sepsis. Critical Care Medicine 1992;20:864-874

ANSWER 52

A. FALSE   B. TRUE   C. TRUE   D. TRUE   E. FALSE

AST = Aspartate aminotransferase. ALT = Alanine aminotransferase. ALP = Alkaline phosphatase. Qualitative tests of liver function can be divided into markers for hepatic damage, cholestasis and reduced synthetic function. Hepatic damage: AST occurs in many tissues and is therefore less liver specific but is more sensitive than ALT in indicating liver damage. Lactate dehydrogenase is also insensitive although isoenzyme electrophoresis may help in distinguishing liver damage. Glutamate dehydrogenase increases when liver damage is predominantly centrilobular. Cholestasis: Bilirubin levels rise in haemolysis, liver cell damage and biliary tract obstruction. Biliary obstruction typically shows an increase in the conjugated fraction. ALP rises in pregnancy, bone disease and biliary tract obstruction. Gamma-glutamyl transferase is very sensitive for both hepatic and biliary disease. Synthetic function: Albumin concentrations decrease in acute illnesses largely due to protein metabolism. Cholinesterase activity falls in patients with severe liver damage. Transferrin, caeruloplasmin, thyroid binding globulin, alpha-2 antitrypsin and pseudocholinesterase may also fall. Most coagulation factors are synthesised in the liver and have a short half life, so their measurement may be useful in detecting liver damage. However, coagulation may be normal despite loss of significant functional liver.

Ref: Roe PG. Liver function tests in the critically ill patient. Clinical Intensive care 1993;4:174-182

ANSWER 53

A. FALSE   B. TRUE   C. TRUE   D. TRUE   E. TRUE

The APACHE (acute physiology and chronic health evaluation) II classification was described in 1985 as a refinement of the original APACHE. APACHE III was described in 1991. APACHE II is designed and validated to be measured using the worst physiological variables from the first 24 hours of a patients stay in the ICU. Variables measured are temperature, mean arterial pressure, heart rate, respiratory rate, oxygenation, arterial pH, serum sodium, potassium and creatinine, haematocrit, white cell count and Glasgow Coma Score. Each variable scores between 0 and 4 points depending on the extent of derangement. Points are also added for age and a history of severe organ system insufficiency or immunocompromise. The resulting score is the APACHE II score. This score can be entered into an equation that also includes weighting for diagnostic category and post-emergency surgery to compute death rates for groups of acutely ill patients. It should not be used for individual predictions.

Ref: Knaus WA, Draper EA, Wagner DP, Zimmerman JE. APACHE II: A severity of disease classification system. Critical Care Medicine 1985;13:818-829

ANSWER 54

A. TRUE   B. FALSE   C. FALSE   D. TRUE   E. TRUE

Complications relating to the catheter are the commonest, including pneumothorax, vessel perforation, thrombosis, embolisation of air or catheter and most importantly infection. Fluid overload is common, particularly in the elderly. Hyperosmolar dehydration syndrome occurs if hyperglycaemia is allowed to occur. Persistent glycosuria and / or an osmotic diuresis are warning signs. The blood glucose level should be kept below 11 mmol/l. Electrolyte imbalances may occur, particularly hypokalaemia, hypomagnesaemia & hypophosphataemia. Metabolic acidosis may occur from the amino acid solutions used due to a large amount of hydrochlorides, a high titratable acidity or an excess of cationic amino acids which produce an excess of H^+ ions when metabolised. Essential fatty acid deficiency may occur if lipid free TPN is used. Rebound hypoglycaemia may occur if TPN is suddenly stopped due to the high levels of endogenous insulin. Vitamin and trace element deficiencies may occur, in particular folic acid and zinc.

Ref: T.E. OH. Intensive Care Manual. Butterworths. Third Edition. Ch 82. Parenteral Nutrition

ANSWER 55

A. FALSE   B. TRUE   C. FALSE   D. TRUE   E. TRUE

The diagnosis of brain stem death has a few preconditions:

The patient must be in apnoeic coma.

There should be no metabolic derangements.

Primary hypothermia must be excluded.

There should be no effects of drugs contributing to the condition eg sedatives, opiates, relaxants.

There should be no doubt that the patient's condition is due to irremediable structural brain damage.

The time of the first test is recommended to be delayed until at least 24 hours following a hypoxic cardiac arrest but can be tested earlier after an obvious primary head injury eg 4-6 hours. If a patient carries a signed donor card, or has otherwise recorded his wishes, there is no legal requirement to establish lack of objection on the part of the relatives, although it is good practice to take account of the views of close relatives. As far as is known no major religious grouping in the UK objects to the principle of organ donation. The Jehovah's Witnesses have religious objections to blood tranfusion, but feel that donating or receiving organs is a matter for each member to decide for themself. Doll's eyes reflex is not part of the brain stem reflexes tested to confirm death.

Ref: BMJ 1982; 285: pg 1558-60 & pg 1641-4. Diagnosis of brain stem death I & II. HMSO 1983. Cadaveric organs for transplantation. A code of practice including the diagnosis of brain death.

ANSWER 56

A. TRUE   B. FALSE   C. TRUE   D. FALSE   E. FALSE

Neuronal dysfunction occurs within seconds of the onset of cerebral ischaemia. Within 6 to 8 minutes permanent neuronal injury has occurred. Haemodilution can improve cerebral blood flow and oxygen delivery to the ischaemic area surrounding the infarcted tissue. Nimodipine has been shown to reduce delayed cerebral ischaemia following aneurysmal subarachnoid haemorrhage, but is not of benefit to those suffering acute ischaemic stroke. Tirilizad mesylate is a 21-aminosteroid that does not possess glucocorticoid activity but is a potent lipid peroxidase inhibitor and free radical scavenger. The indications for its use are not as yet defined. N-methyl-D-aspartate calcium channels have been implicated as the cause of the high intracellular calcium concentrations during ischaemia/reperfusion injury. Antagonists are therefore under trial but, again, indications for their use are awaited.

Ref: Klebanoff LM. An update on ischaemic stroke. Current Opinion in Critical Care 1995;1:89-97

ANSWER   57

A. FALSE   B. FALSE   C. FALSE   D. FALSE   E. TRUE

GBS is an inflammatory demyelinating polyneuropathy that is antibody mediated. It often occurs as an aberrant response to a viral illness (60% of cases). Typically there is a progressive and symmetrical ascending flaccid motor paralysis following paraesthesia of the extremities. Tendon reflexes are absent and muscle pain is common. Progressive weakness may cause respiratory failure, glottic incompetence and ophthalmoplegia. Fisher's variant describes ophthalmoplegia, ataxia and areflexia with little weakness. Although the CSF may have a raised protein concentration, it may be normal (particularly early in the course) and is not diagnostic. The diagnosis is clinical, often supported with nerve conduction studies demonstrating demyelination. Treatment includes airway protection and assisted ventilation together with general support e.g. enteral feeding, physiotherapy, venous thrombosis prophylaxis. Autonomic dysfunction may result in cardiac dysrhythmias, hyper and hypotension. Plasmapheresis should be performed early to be of benefit. There is evidence that intravenous immune globulin is also effective, and may be equally efficacious. The schedule for both treatments is not precisely defined. With good medical and nursing care, most patients recover within 6 months. However, 65% have minor problems, 5-10% have significant deficits and 5% develop a relapsing form of the disease.

Ref: Hillman and Bishop. Clinical Intensive Care. Cambridge University Press. Ch 26

ANSWER   58

A. FALSE   B. FALSE   C. FALSE   D. TRUE   E. FALSE

Chest tube drainage is indicated for removing gas, blood, serous fluid, lymph or GI contents from the pleural space. Some pneumothoraces may be treated conservatively if they are small and not causing cardio-respiratory embarrassment. Alternatively, aspiration of a simple pneumothorax is sometimes recommended. Chest tube drainage should follow needle thoracostomy if a tension pneumothorax is present. If a penetrating injury to the chest is present, the entry site should be avoided. Infection is more likely and the wound may need exploration (it may also not lie immediately over the pleural space). The normal landmarks are either the 5th/6th intercostal space in the mid axillary line or the 2nd intercostal space in the mid clavicular line. Following skin cleansing and LA infiltration, the skin is incised and blunt dissection to the pleural cavity is performed. The track should pass immediately above a rib to avoid the neurovascular bundle that runs on each ribs inferior border. A finger is pushed into the pleural cavity to feel for any viscus that may be injured and the chest tube is inserted with forceps (not the sharp trochar that some drains are presented with). This is then connected to a one way valve and sutured in position. If more than 1.5-2 litres of blood drains, or the ongoing loss is greater than 200 mls/hr (in an adult), this suggests the need for surgical review and possible thoracotomy.

Ref: Baskett, Dow, Nolan, Maull. Practical Procedures in Anesthesia and Critical Care. Mosby. Ch 2.

ANSWER 59

A. TRUE   B. TRUE   C. TRUE   D. TRUE   E. TRUE

The optimal time to protect the kidneys from an insult is before it happens. The cells which are particularly susceptible are those in the ascending loop of Henle as they are so metabolically active and these are among the cells to be worst affected in ATN. Common potential precipitants of acute renal failure include major surgery, IV contrast agents, nephrotoxic drugs, rhabdomyolysis and tumour lysis. Rhabdomyoloysis sufficient to cause ATN may follow crush injury, burns, seizures, muscle infarction and diabetic ketoacidosis. Acute intravascular haemolysis can also result in ATN and may occur in transfusion reactions, severe falciparum malaria, thrombotic microangiopathy and G-6-PD deficiency.

Ref: British Journal of Hospital Medicine 1996; Vol 55, No 4: pg 162-166. Prevention of acute renal failure.

ANSWER 60

A. FALSE   B. TRUE   C. TRUE   D. FALSE   E. TRUE

Cardiogenic shock is shock caused by heart disease and is defined as a systolic blood pressure < 90 mmHg with evidence of reduced blood flow as shown by :-

Urine output < 20 ml/hr

Impaired mental function

Peripheral vasoconstriction with cold, clammy skin

Other changes seen include reduced coronary blood flow, myocardial lactate production, high myocardial oxygen extraction, and an intense neurohumoral stress response.

Autopsies have shown that over 40% of functioning myocardium has been lost in patients who die of cardiogenic shock after MI. Most patients with cardiogenic shock have elevated LVEDP and PCWP, but PCWP may not be elevated as a result of fluid lost into the lungs, diuretic therapy, relative hypovolaemia, or right ventricular infarction. IABP should be considered for patients who remain hypotensive and shocked after a short trial of aggressive medical therapy. The IABP is contra-indicated in patients with aortic regurgitation.

Ref: T.E. OH. Intensive Care Manual. Butterworths. 3rd Ed. Ch 59. Cardiogenic Shock

ANSWER 61

A. FALSE   B. FALSE   C. TRUE   D. FALSE   E. TRUE

Serum potassium levels are governed both by internal and external potassium balance. Internal potassium balance refers to uptake or loss of potassium from cells. Uptake, via the Na-K-ATPase pump, is stimulated by insulin and beta-adrenergic stimulation. Potassium loss from cells is stimulated by acidosis, alpha-adrenergic stimulation and cell damage. Heparin can stimulate the decreased secretion of aldosterone which is involved with renal potassium excretion and external potassium balance.

Ref: Current Anaesthesia and Critical Care 1996; Vol 7, No 4: pg 176-181. Physiology and pathophysiology of fluid and electrolytes.

ANSWER 62

A. TRUE   B. TRUE   C. FALSE   D. FALSE   E. TRUE

DVT and PE are common complications of major trauma. A recent study found a DVT incidence of 58% in the lower legs. More than 80% of the patients with spinal cord trauma had DVT, and two of the three fatal pulmonary emboli in this study (349 patients) were in patients with spinal cord trauma. Early fracture fixation reduces the incidence of ARDS, fat embolism and mortality. Glutamine is the preferred nutrient of the enterocyte and should be given to all enterally fed patients except those with the possibility of cerebral ischaemia as it is metabolised/converted to glutamate, an inhibitory neurotransmitter which may worsen cerebral outcome. Up to 80% of patients staying 5 days or more on ITU become colonized with potentially pathogenic micro-organisms. In trauma patients hypothermia correlates with poor survival such that those with a core temperature dropping below 34 degrees centigrade have 40% mortality compared with 7% mortality for those whose lowest recorded temperature is 34 degrees or above.

Ref: Current Anaesthesia and Critical Care 1996; Vol 7, No 3: pg 139-145 Care for trauma patients in the intensive care unit

ANSWER 63

A. TRUE   B. TRUE   C. TRUE   D. FALSE   E. TRUE

The actual incidence of PE is difficult to assess but autopsy reports have indicated that 15% of deaths are directly attributable to PE. The classic S1Q3 T3 ECG is not often seen. The commonest findings are those representing right heart strain. Embolization of bone marrow (fat embolism), tumour (choriocarcinoma, renal vein tumour), air and amniotic fluid can all result in pulmonary artery occlusion. A high mortality is associated with major air and amniotic fluid embolism. Anticoagulation may be required following air embolism to prevent thrombus forming around residual intra-cardiopulmonary air bubbles.

Ref: T.E. OH. Intensive Care Manual.Butterworths. 3rd Ed. Ch 26. Pulmonary embolism.

ANSWER 64

A. TRUE   B. TRUE   C. FALSE   D. TRUE   E. TRUE

Lactic acid is a weak acid that is completely dissociated at normal pH (pKa 3.8). Apart from the red cell (which lacks mitochondria), pyruvate can be metabolised to acetyl-CoA, alanine and alpha-keto-glutarate, but in a reaction catalysed by lactate dehydrogenase it can also be converted to lactate. The liver usually clears half of the lactate production, most of the remainder being metabolised and/or excreted by the kidneys. Normal blood lactate is approximately 1 mmol/l. Increased levels are either due to inadequate tissue perfusion (Type A = acute circulatory failure, shock, hypoxia, anaemia or increased oxygen consumption) or metabolic derangements (Type B = neoplastic disease, diabetes, vitamin deficiency, ethanol intoxication, biguanides and inborn errors of metabolism including type 1 glycogen storage disease, fructose 1,6 diphosphate deficiency and pyruvate dehydrogenase deficiency). Hyperlactatemia in the critically ill is usually a marker of tissue hypoxia. Treatment is of the underlying cause. The acidosis produced is not routinely treated with bicarbonate as intracellular acidosis may worsen, but this is controversial.

Ref: Bakker J. Monitoring of blood lactate levels. International Journal of Intensive Care 1996;3:29-36

ANSWER   65

A. FALSE   B. TRUE   C. FALSE   D. FALSE   E. TRUE

DIC occurs when the balance of the haemostatic and fibrinolytic systems become mismatched. It is characterized by intravascular consumption of clotting factors and platelets resulting in varying degrees of microvascular obstruction. The clinical presentation varies with patients showing thrombotic, haemorrhagic or mixed manifestations. The definitive treatment is of the underlying cause with appropriate supportive management. Laboratory finding may include various combinations of prolonged TT, PT/INR, APTT; hypofibrinogenaemia; thrombocytopaenia; low factor VIII; and excess fibrinolysis with elevated FDPs. Cryoprecipitate is obtained by thawing FFP at 4 degrees centigrade and contains concentrated factor VIII and fibrinogen. The use of heparin in DIC is controversial but if used the starting doses should be small eg 50 - 100 units/kg, followed by 10-15 units/kg/hr.

Ref: T.E. OH. Intensive Care Manual. Butterworths. 3rd Ed. Ch 88 Haemostatic Failure.

ANSWER   66

A. FALSE   B. FALSE   C. FALSE   D. TRUE   E. TRUE

Sodium bicarbonate has been used in the treatment of metabolic acidoses for over 50 years and until recently has been a matter of routine. Theoretically sodium bicarbonate should react with the hydrogen ion from an organic acid resulting in the formation of the sodium salt, water and carbon dioxide. However when there is metabolic acidosis in the presence of tissue hypoxia the available tissue oxygen is not sufficient for the individual's metabolic needs. Administration of bicarbonate will tend to further limit the available oxygen, via the Bohr effect, increase lactate production and thus worsen the acidosis. However, if the metabolic acidosis is not associated with tissue hypoxia, bicarbonate may raise the arterial pH and be beneficial. In fact, in patients with renal tubular acidosis, diarrhoea or uraemic acidosis the arterial pH generally improves with the administration of sodium bicarbonate. There are several potential negative effects of bicarbonate administration:- Venous hypercapnia with an increased mixed venous carbon dioxide content leading to a fall in tissue pH, fall in CSF pH, tissue hypoxia, circulatory congestion/overload, hypernatraemia.

Some patients with diabetic ketoacidosis or hepatic failure have impaired tissue oxygen delivery and the above complications can be observed therefore bicarbonate treatment should be avoided. Similarly tissue oxygen delivery is impaired and is an important cause of lactate accumulation in patients following drowning, cardiac arrest, circulatory shock and sepsis. The administration of sodium bicarbonate does not improve the underlying tissue hypoxia or clinical outcome.

Ref: Current Anaesthesia and Critical Care 1996; Vol 7, No 4: pg 182-186. Current concepts in acid-base balance: use of bicarbonate in patients with metabolic acidosis.

ANSWER   67

A. TRUE   B. FALSE   C. TRUE   D. FALSE   E. TRUE

Central venous catheter related infection is the most common life-threatening complication of their use. The rate of septicaemia associated with CVCs is 4-14%.

Proven techniques for reducing infection include;

  i) Skilled teams to insert and maintain the catheters (the incidence is reduced 5-8 times)

 ii) Sterile gloves, gown, cap, mask and a large drape (a sixfold reduction)

iii) Topical disinfectants (2% chlorhexidine is more effective than 10% povidone iodine or 70%

alcohol). Antibiotic containing solutions may also reduce infection rates, but fungal infections may be favoured.

iv) Silver impregnated cuff (this reduces short term infection rates, but does not reduce infection in long term tunnelled catheters).

v) Flushing catheters with an antibiotic/antithrombotic combination (although this reduces colonisation, its effects on bacteraemia and the emergence of resistance is unknown).

vi) A hub connector that results in sterilisation of an infusion needle using iodine each time it is connected can reduce the incidence 4 times.

vii) Antimicrobial coating of catheters (particularly if both external and internal surfaces are treated).

Exchange over a guidewire may result in transfer of organisms to the new catheter. If this method is used, then quantitative culture of the removed catheter and blood culture surveillance should be considered.

Ref: Raad I, Darouiche R. Prevention of infections associated with intravascular devices. Current Opinion in Critical Care 1996;2:361-365

ANSWER 68

A. TRUE   B. TRUE   C. TRUE   D. TRUE   E. FALSE

Inhalational injury should be suspected if there is a history of exposure to smoke, particularly if it occurred in a confined space or there is a reduced conscious level. It should be suspected if there is hoarseness, cough and sooty sputum, singed nasal hairs, facial burns or mucosal injury to the mouth or pharynx. It is best documented by fibreoptic bronchoscopy and a CXR is of little help initially as positive findings appear late. Similarly arterial blood gases and SpO_2 may appear normal in the event of carbon monoxide intoxication despite significant levels of carboxyhaemoglobin. However, co-oximetry can differentiate COHb from oxyhaemoglobin.

Careful observation is required following an inhalational injury as severe airway obstruction can develop after a 'free period' of 3-8 hours. Some authors advocate prophylactic tracheal intubation. Whilst there is no benefit in prophylactic antibiotic or steroid therapy, steroids may be required along with aminophylline if severe bronchospasm develops. Enteral feeding has been shown to protect against gut translocation of toxins and micro-orgainsms and to reduce the incidence of sepsis. SDD does not improve survival in burnt patients, unlike in trauma victims, but it may reduce the incidence of pulmonary infections.

Ref: Current Anaesthesia and Critical Care. 1996; Vol 7, No 1: pg 31 - 36. Intensive care treatment of burn patients.

ANSWER 69

A. FALSE   B. TRUE   C. TRUE   D. FALSE   E. FALSE

Hospital wide pneumonia ranks second to urinary tract infection as the most common nosocomial infection. In ICU's it accounts for almost ½ of infections, whereas blood stream infections only accounted for 12%. Diagnosis is often difficult as fever, leucocytosis, purulent secretions and radiographic abnormalities may occur in other conditions. Endotracheal aspirates identify most pathogens but may show colonising organisms. Bronchoscopic protected specimen brush (PSB), bronchoalveolar lavage (BAL) and non-bronchoscopic BAL have been studied, but as yet their role remains unclear. Pseudomonas aeriginosa infection is more common in those undergoing prolonged ventilation, with chronic lung disease, or having received prior antibiotics or corticosteroids. Staphylococcus aureus is more common in those suffering from coma, diabetes mellitus, head trauma, renal failure or influenza. Nosocomial pneumonia occurring within 4 days of hospital admission tend to be due to Staphylococcus aureus, Streptococcus pneumoniae and Haemophilus influenzae, whereas those acquired after this are more commonly due to gram -ve bacteria.

Ref: Cassiere HA, Niederman MS. Diagnosis and treatment of nosocomial pneumonia. Current Opinion in Critical Care 1996;2:22-28

ANSWER   70

A. FALSE   B. TRUE   C. TRUE   D. TRUE   E. FALSE

Tetanus is caused by the anaerobic gram positive rod Clostridium tetani, the spores of which are found in animal faeces, on the ground and in the soil. It produces tetanospasmin and tetanolysin- both exotoxins. The former diffuses from the infected site via the alpha motor neurones cell bodies to many areas of the spinal cord and brain stem. Here it inhibits the release of glycine and GABA, the inhibitory neurotransmitters, resulting in increases in muscle tone, muscle spasm and autonomic instability. Tetanolysin reduces wound viability of the infected site. Clinical features are muscle rigidity and spasms, dysphagia, laryngospasm and autonomic instability (most commonly hypertension and tachydysrhythmias). Shorter incubation and onset of symptoms, and autonomic instability carry a worse prognosis. Treatment includes securing the airway urgently, rehydration (salivation may result in large fluid losses), wound debridement and penicillin/metronidazole/human tetanus immunoglobulin treatment. Heavy sedation with benzodiazepines, barbiturates and phenothiazines result in reduction of muscle spasms and autonomic instability. Neuromuscular blockade may be required in initial control but will mask inadequate sedation and therefore should not be used routinely.

Ref: Linton DM. Acute neurological disorders: perioperative and critical care management strategies. Current Anaesrthesia and Critical Care 1992;3:162-167.

ANSWER   71

A. TRUE   B. FALSE   C. TRUE   D. FALSE   E. FALSE

Human malignant hyperthermia is inherited as an autosomal dominant condition with links to gene loci on chromosomes 17 and 19. Triggering agents include suxamethonium, (which can produce a very rapid onset) halothane, enflurane, isoflurane, desflurane, sevoflurane, methoxyflurane, ether and cyclopropane. The incidence is approximately 1/15,000 anaesthetics. Mannitol is present in bottles of Dantrolene to make the solution isotonic. Miller suggests that 3-4 people will be needed to get a dose of 2gm/kg into solution for an adult. Even in high dose, dantrolene will only produce mild muscle weakness.

Ref: Miller. Anesthesia. Churchill Livingstone. Chapter 31.

ANSWER   72

A. FALSE   B. TRUE   C. FALSE   D. FALSE   E. FALSE

This question requires a 5/5 answer. Be sure to revise the protocols the night before the exam, defects in resuscitation knowledge are a recipe for disaster. The massage to ventilation ratio is 15 : 2. The dose of atropine in asystole is 3 mg given once only and 5 mg of adrenaline is given after 3 cycles if there is no response.

Ref: BNF. September 1996. p103

ANSWER   73
A. FALSE   B. FALSE   C. TRUE   D. FALSE   E. TRUE

There is an international colour code for cylinder contents (oxygen, white; nitrous oxide, blue; air, white and black) however it is not used in a number of countries. The filling ratio for nitrous oxide is less in the tropics to prevent too high a pressure developing in cylinders. The pin index system applies up to size E cylinders

Ref. Dorsch & Dorsch. Understanding anaesthetic equipment: Construction, Care and Complications. Chapter 1: Compressed gas cylinders.
Ref. Craft & Upton. Key topics in anaesthesia. Carbon dioxide. Oxygen. Nitrous oxide.

ANSWER   74
A. FALSE   B. TRUE   C. FALSE   D. TRUE   E. FALSE

Indicators in CO_2 absorbers can be confusing since phenolphthalein is white when fresh and pink on exhaustion. Mimosa Z is correspondingly red and then white. If the fresh gas flow is upstream of the absorber, anaesthetic agent may be retained in the absorber, especially during induction. Also the vapouriser should be downstream of the absorber to reduce moisture condensing in the vapouriser and to reduce vapour loss during induction prior to reaching the patient. Resistance rises with increased respiratory rate. A fresh gas flow of greater than 5 lpm only marginally increases the speed of denitrogenation.

Ref. Dorsch & Dorsch Understanding anaesthetic equipment: Construction, Care and Complications. Chapter 8. The breathing system. IV The Circle System

ANSWER   75
A. FALSE   B. FALSE   C. FALSE   D. TRUE   E. TRUE

In 1977 Goldmann published an index of risk of cardiac mortality following non-cardiac surgery. Presence of the following result in a positive score: Heart failure (11); MI within 6 months (10), ECG rhythm not sinus (7), ECG >5 VEs/min (7), Age >70 (5), Emergency op (4), Aortic stenosis (3), Intra-thoracic /intra-abdominal /aortic surgery (3), Concurrent respiratory disease /renal disease /hepatic disease /hypokalaemia /acidosis (3).

Ref: Nimmo & Smith. Anaesthesia Vol 1. Ch25. (Blackwell).

ANSWER   76
A. FALSE   B. TRUE   C. FALSE   D. TRUE   E. FALSE

Brief general anaesthesia is necessary for ECT. Methohexitone or propofol should be used and suxamethonium is given to prevent injuries during the convulsion.

Ref: Yentis, Hirsch, and Smith. Anaesthesia A-Z. pp156

ANSWER 77

A. FALSE   B. FALSE   C. TRUE   D. FALSE   E. TRUE

Nerve roots C1–C3 need to be blocked to perform CEA under local, it has the advantage of continuous neurological monitoring. Isoflurane is the agent of choice as it is associated with a lower critical regional blood flow. EEG monitoring has not been proved to improve outcome.

Ref: Miller. Anaesthesia 4th ed.

ANSWER 78

A. FALSE   B. TRUE   C. TRUE   D. TRUE   E. TRUE

The QT interval is measured from the beginning of the QRS to the end of the T wave. It does not relate to atrial contraction, being the length of ventricular contraction. It is corrected for heart rate by dividing by the square root of the preceeding R-R interval. It is shortened by digoxin therapy, hyperkalaemia and hypercalcaemia.

Ref. Yentis, Hirsch & Smith. Anaesthesia A to Z. Butterworth Heinemann. QT interval. Torsade de Pointes.

ANSWER 79

A. TRUE   B. TRUE   C. FALSE   D. FALSE   E. TRUE

Bladder sensation is carried up to T9 and regional blockade to this level is recommended. There is no difference in mortality, morbidity, or cognitive function after TURP with either regional or general anaesthesia. TUR syndrome occurs as irrigation fluid enters the venous circulation by hydrostatic pressure (increased incidence using drip stands >60cm above the patient and in a head down position). The absorbed fluid expands the intravascular volume and dilutes the ECF electrolytes. Under GA, features of hypervolaemia present initially, whereas under regional anaesthesia the features of hyponatraemia are more likely to appear first

Ref: Bernstein S. Regional anaesthesia for urological surgery. Int Anes Clinics 31.pp 57-66 Nimmo & Smith. Anaesthesia - Vol 1. (Blackwell). pp372

ANSWER 80

A. FALSE   B. TRUE   C. FALSE   D. TRUE   E. TRUE

Anaemia is the result of a 50% plasma expansion as compared to a 20% red cell expansion. T wave changes and left axis deviation are commom and result from diaphragmatic displacement. The increased MV is a central progesterone effect. The reduced FRC and raised oxygen consumption during pregnancy increase the risks of anaesthesia.

Ref: Yentis, Hirsch, Smith. Anaesthesia A-Z. Butterworths. pp 367

ANSWER 81

A. FALSE   B. TRUE   C. FALSE   D. TRUE   E. FALSE

Sickle cell disease is commonest in people originating in west and central afrIca and also from around the mediterranean. Sickle cell trait is present in 10% of African Americans in whom 40% of their Hb is as HbS. Sickle cell anaemia is found in 1% of African Americans and their Hb is very predominantly HbS. On desaturation of their Hb the HbS is 50 times less soluble than HbA and tactoids of rigid Hb chains are formed altering the function of the red blood cells. Haemolytic anaemia occurs along with organ damage due to to vascular obstruction in the spleen, kidneys, gut, and brain. Aplastic crises can occur when the bone marrow fails as a result of intercurrent infection or folate deficiency. Exchange transfusion is appropriate prior to major vascular surgery as O_2 carriage is increased and the risk of sickling is decreased. Folate therapy is appropriate as it may help marrow function at a time of additional stress. Esmarch tourniquets have been described as used without problems in some patients although overall the use of tourniquets would be considered contra-indicated.

Ref: Katz J. Anaesthesia and uncommon diseases. Saunders. Sickle cell anaemia. p391-397.

ANSWER 82

A. TRUE   B. FALSE   C. FALSE   D. FALSE   E. TRUE

All halogenated agents impair hypoxic pulmonary vasoconstriction (HPV) in vitro, isoflurane has been shown to have a dose dependent effect in vivo. Ketamine is a safe agent as it provides anaesthesia, analgesia and has no effect on HPV. During single lung ventilation there is a 20-60% decrease in blood flow to the nondependent lung which leads to a right to left shunt. Only after the chest is open does mediastinal shift and motion impair ventilation and the circulation.

Ref: Miller RD. Anesthesia 3rd ed. Churchill Livingstone. Ch50 pp 1533-1537

ANSWER 83

A. FALSE   B. TRUE   C. FALSE   D. FALSE   E. TRUE

During the first stage of labour contraction pains are transmitted via T11 and T12 and experienced in the hypogastrium. Low backache may arise from periuterine structures via the lumbrosacral plexus (L5-S1). During the second stage, pain from the cervix and perineum is transmitted via S234. Therefore, a block up to T10 and down to the sacral roots will be required to prevent pain from uterine contractions and a dilating cervix. Nitrous oxide is useful in up to 50% of cases, 30% receive no benefit. The epidural space volume is reduced by engorged veins. Pethidine may cause neonatal respiratory depression within 2 hours of delivery.

Ref: Yentis, Hirsch, and Smith. Anaesthesia A-Z. Butterworths. pp 328

ANSWER 84

A. FALSE   B. FALSE   C. FALSE   D. FALSE   E. TRUE

Mediastinal masses lead to compression of airway, heart and the superior vena cava. The airway is the structure most commonly obstructed and lymphoma is the usual cause. Compression of the superior vena cava is usually by a bronchial carcinoma. Direct compression of the heart is much less common than that of airway or superior vena cava. If respiratory symptoms are present with superior vena cava compression they are usually due to distended veins compressing the airway or due to airway oedema.

Ref: Miller Anesthesia. Chapter 52. Anaesthesia for thoracic surgery.

ANSWER   85

A. TRUE   B. FALSE   C. FALSE   D. FALSE   E. TRUE

Arterial blood gas analysis during hypothermia is either with temperature compensation (pH-stat) or without compensation (alpha-stat). Gas solubility increases as temperature drops so using temperature compensation to the patients core temperature will measure a lower $PaCO_2$ than without. If pH-stat management is used then CO_2 may be added to maintain a 'normal' pH. Cerebral blood flow autoregulation is maintained using alpha-stat management so this is most commonly used for adult hypothermic bypass. Aprotinin inhibits fibrinolysis by inhibiting plasmin. As a part of the stress response, glucagon is released and there is an inhibition of the effects of insulin on glucose homeostasis. Ventricular fibrillation as 'myocardial preservation' prevents the need for any crystalloid cardioplegia to return to the cardiopulmonary bypass circuit so reducing haemodilution.

Ref: Hensley FA Jnr. The practice of cardiac anaesthesia. Chapters 20.

ANSWER   86

A. FALSE   B. TRUE   C. TRUE   D. TRUE   E. FALSE

Air embolus is likely to occur via large veins or venous sinuses if the intravascular pressure becomes negative. Venous pressure can be raised by volume loading, reduction of venous capacitance, maintenance of positive intrathoracic pressure and alterations in posture. Following diagnosis of air embolus, management is aimed at limiting further entrainment by flooding the surgical field and raising venous pressure, preventing expansion by switching off nitrous oxide if used, whilst attempting to retain the embolus in the atrium (lateral position) where it may be possible to aspirate it via a central venous catheter.

Ref: Yentis, Hirsch, and Smith. Anaesthesia A-Z. Butterworths. pp10

ANSWER   87

A. TRUE   B. TRUE   C. FALSE   D. FALSE   E. FALSE

Monitoring with the standard three electrode system only allows leads I, II, and III to be monitored, this will not allow anterior ischaemia to be detected. The 5 electrode system allows all 6 standard limb leads to be recorded along with one precordial lead, 90% of episodes of ischaemia will be detected. The modified 3 lead system can be as sensitive as the standard V5 monitoring in picking up episodes of ischaemia. In the CM5 three lead system the right arm electrode goes on the manubrium and this monitoring is particularly good for assessing anterior ischaemia.

Ref. Hensley. The practice of cardiac anaesthesia. Monitoring the cardiac surgical patient.

ANSWER 88

A. FALSE   B. FALSE   C. FALSE   D. TRUE   E. TRUE

The classification of ventilators is complex. There is Ward's system of mechanical thumbs, minute volume dividers, bag squeezers, and intermittent blowers. There is Mapleson's division on the basis of the characteristics of inspiration and the cycling from inspiration to expiration. Pressure generators only produce low pressures with a marked dependence of tidal volume on airway resistance and overall compliance. Flow generators which give a higher inspiratory pressure can have constant or non-constant flows. There is overlap in this classification of ventilators since some ventilators (The Servo) can operate in either fashion. Jetting devices work at pressures of up to 4 bar and although most of the Manleys are minute volume dividers the 'Servovent' is a bag squeezer.

Ref: Ward. Anaesthetic equipment. Chapter 11. Resuscitators and automatic ventilators.
Ref: Yentis, Hirsch & Smith. Anaesthesia A to Z. Ventilators.

ANSWER 89

A. FALSE   B. FALSE   C. FALSE   D. TRUE   E. TRUE

Pain is subjective and its severity is widely variable and is difficult to predict. Pain scoring includes the use of scales such as the visual analogue scale (VAS). This has been found reliable in children over the age of 5. The Magill Pain Questionnaire is a development that allows description of both character and severity of pain by adjectival description. In children although the gold standard for pain assessment is self-reporting this may be misleading. Post-operative pain may be denied for fear of an injection. Other methods of pain assessment in children include behavioral and biological measures. The latter include palmar sweating which has been found to be a successful index of pain in heel lancing.

Refs: Melzack, R. and Katz, J. (1994) Pain measurement in persons in pain. In: Wall, P.D. and Melzack, R. (Eds.) Textbook of Pain, 3rd edn. pp. 337-356. Edinburgh: Churchill Livingstone and McGrath, P.J. and Unruh, A.M. (1994) Measurement and assessment of paediatric pain. In: Wall, P.D. and Melzack, R. (Eds.) Textbook of Pain, 3rd edn. pp. 303-314. Edinburgh: Churchill Livingstone

ANSWER 90

A. TRUE   B. TRUE   C. FALSE   D. FALSE   E. TRUE

Chassaignac's tubercle, the transverse process of C6, is the most prominent landmark used for correct siting of a stellate ganglion block. It can be found by sliding a finger posterolaterally from the cricoid cartilage whilst displacing the carotid artery laterally. A successful block is associated with a Horners syndrome (small pupil, anhydrosis, ptosis) and nasal and conjunctival congestion. Complications include intravascular injection (NB vertebral artery), recurrent laryngeal nerve block, phrenic nerve block and epidural or subarachnoid injection. Brachial plexus blockade and haematomas may also occur.

Ref: Miller RD. Anesthesia. Ch46. (Churchill Livingstone).

Exam 3

QUESTION 1

Propofol

A. Is contraindicated in patients with porphyria
B. Causes pain on intravenous injection in less than 5% of patients
C. 25% is excreted unchanged in the urine
D. Has a volume of distribution at steady state greater than 250 litres
E. May safely be mixed with alfentanil for combined administration

QUESTION 2

In the management of a patient for an awake intubation

A. The maximum recommended dose of cocaine for surface tissue use is 1.5mg/kg
B. The superior laryngeal nerve is a branch of the glossopharyngeal nerve
C. A glossopharyngeal nerve block risks airway obstruction
D. Superior laryngeal nerve block can be achieved by placing anaesthetic in the piriform fossae
E. For a transtracheal approach local anaesthetic must be injected during expiration

QUESTION 3

In patients that present for neurosurgical procedures

A. The normal intracranial pressure is 0-10 mmHg
B. ICP is equal to mean arterial pressure minus cerebral perfusion pressure
C. A III nerve palsy is a sign of tentorial coning in a patient with raised ICP
D. Medullary coning may present as decerebrate rigidity
E. An ICP of 15-20 mmHg requires active treatment

QUESTION 4

Direct arterial pressure waveform

A. The systolic pressure measured in the dorsalis pedis artery is about 20 mmHg less than that in the radial artery
B. The mean arterial pressure measured peripherally is similar to that measured centrally
C. A low 'shoulder' to the waveform suggests hypovolaemia
D. In spontaneous respiration the arterial pressure falls during inspiration
E. The trace seen from the radial artery has a dicrotic notch

QUESTION 5

In the preoperative assessment of the adult airway

A. Mallampati class 2 assessment includes a visible uvula
B. Distance between the mandible and hyoid bones should ideally be less than 2 finger-breadths
C. A Mallampati grade 3 airway is classified using a standard laryngoscope blade
D. Patients with sarcoidosis should be considered at risk of airway obstruction
E. The patient with scleroderma is more likely to have an abnormal airway

QUESTION 6

Respiratory Function tests

A. Increased functional residual capacity (FRC) suggests restrictive disease
B. Reduced maximum voluntary ventilation (MVV) is a poor predictor of post-operative complications
C. A predicted post-operative FEV1 of > 800 ml is associated with a successful outcome after surgery
D. A reduced FEV1 implies an obstructive defect
E. Assessment of closing capacity will display the early effects of smoking

QUESTION 7

When monitoring intracranial pressure

A. The waveform obtained resembles an arterial waveform
B. A ventricular drain is least prone to infection as it is placed during craniotomy
C. A pressure of over 30 mm Hg requires active management
D. A transducer placed within the brain tissue cannot be used
E. A subarachnoid screw may be placed via a burr hole

QUESTION 8

Concerning the intensive care management of a burned patient during the first week after his injury

A. If 100 Kg with 50% burns his daily caloric need is 3000 kcal
B. Early tracheostomy should be performed
C. A temperature of 38.5 degrees centigrade necessitates antibiotic therapy
D. Enteral supplementation with omega-3 fatty acids, arginine and nucleotides reduces postoperative catabolism
E. Normocapnia may be an impossible goal

QUESTION 9

Concerning the management of a patient with head injury

A. Benzylisoquoliniums are preferable to steroid relaxants for muscle relaxation
B. About 35% of patients with head injury will be operated on immediately
C. About 20% of patients with a closed head injury ultimately die
D. Artificial hyperventilation may worsen cerebral ischaemia
E. The normal intracranial pressure is 5-15 cm Hg

QUESTION 10

In an adult patient who suffers a cardiac arrest resuscitation guidelines suggest

A. A precordial thump for all unconcious patients
B. If iv access cannot be established all drugs should be given at twice the iv dose endotracheally
C. After one dose of iv adrenaline the intra-cardiac route should be considered
D. The appropriate dose of adrenaline is 10mcg/kg
E. High dose adrenaline (100mcg/kg) is more beneficial in children

QUESTION 11

During anaesthesia for a patient with severe mitral stenosis

A. Sinus rhythm is critical since atrial contraction contributes 60% of ventricular filling
B. If a-v pacing is required a long P-R interval is appropriate
C. Afterload reduction is appropriate even if systemic blood pressure is normal
D. Increased pulmonary vascular resistance is not a likely problem
E. There will often be a marked discrepancy between PA diastolic and PA wedge pressures

QUESTION 12

Arterial blood gas samples

A. Storage at room temperature causes a rise in pH
B. A hypothermic patient will have an inaccurately high PO_2 if temperature-correction is not employed
C. Air bubbles in the sample may lead to a fall in the PCO_2
D. Excessive heparin will cause an inaccurately high pH
E. Storage at room temperature causes a fall in PO_2

QUESTION 13

Circulatory responses to hypovolaemia include

A. A tachycardia due to activation of the Bainbridge reflex
B. A greater release of noradrenaline than adrenaline from the adrenal medulla
C. Aldosterone release due to angiotensin III production
D. A vasopressin induced increased free water absorption
E. Increased atrial natriuretic peptide release in the left atrium

QUESTION 14

Concerning head injury

A. Raised intracranial pressure may lead to hypertension and bradycardia
B. Extradural haematomas are more common than subdural haematomas
C. An extradural haemorrhage is characterised by a lucid interval in the history
D. Haemotympanum is a characteristic finding in basal skull fracture
E. All depressed skull fractures require operative management

QUESTION 15

Which of the following are indications for artificial ventilation in an adult at rest

A. A vital capacity of 10 ml/kg
B. A respiratory rate of >35 bpm
C. An oxygen saturation of 88%
D. An A-a oxygen gradient >300mmHg
E. An FEV1 <75% vital capacity

QUESTION 16

Pressure can be measured using a

A. Bourdon gauge
B. Diaphragm
C. Aneroid gauge
D. Liquid manometer
E. Wet spirometer

QUESTION 17

Clinically proven effective treatment of acute myocardial infarction in the first 48 hours includes

- **A.** Diamorphine
- **B.** Oral beta-blockers
- **C.** Angiotensin-converting enzyme inhibitors
- **D.** Magnesium
- **E.** Nifedipine

QUESTION 18

In a neonate with a tracheo-oesophageal fistula

- **A.** An oesophageal tube should be placed prior to surgery
- **B.** The most likely lesion involves a fistula to the distal oesophagus
- **C.** Associated congenital lesions rarely involve the heart
- **D.** After intubation the bevel of the endotracheal tube should face posteriorly
- **E.** A gastrostomy should be performed prior to the thoracic repair

QUESTION 19

In the utilisation, control and measurement of glucose

- **A.** Glucagon increases blood glucose concentrations within minutes
- **B.** Entry of glucose into muscle cells requires the presence of insulin
- **C.** At plasma glucose concentrations of <20mmol/l glucose will not be lost in the urine
- **D.** Plasma measurement by glucose reagent strips depends on the generation of H_2O_2.
- **E.** Insulin causes glucose which cannot be stored as glycogen to be converted into fatty acids

QUESTION 20

Dystrophica myotonica is characterised by

- **A.** Cataracts
- **B.** Frontal baldness
- **C.** Autosomal recessive inheritance
- **D.** Diabetes mellitus
- **E.** Wasting of temporalis muscle

QUESTION 21

Useful therapy in the management of myasthenia gravis include

A. Prednisolone
B. Physostigmine
C. Azathioprine
D. 3,4-diaminopyridine
E. Gamma Globulin

QUESTION 22

The following drugs are useful secondary analgesics in specific painful conditions

A. Cyproheptadine
B. Calcitonin
C. Baclofen
D. Propranolol
E. Carbamazepine

QUESTION 23

Plasmapheresis is of benefit in the following conditions

A. Tetanus
B. Myasthenia gravis
C. Botulism
D. Salicylate overdose
E. Acute inflammatory polyneuropathy (Guillain Barre syndrome)

QUESTION 24

The pathways of pain sensation include

A. A-delta fibres which terminate in lamina I of the dorsal horn
B. Second order neurones which ascend in the ipsilateral spinothalamic tracts
C. C fibres which release histamine and serotonin
D. Synapses in the substantia nigra of the spinal cord
E. Descending pathways in the dorsolateral columns

QUESTION 25

Concerning congestive cardiac failure

A. Prolonged high dose diuretic therapy reduces afterload
B. Angiotensin converting enzyme (ACE) inhibitors increase cardiac output by 20%
C. Calcium channel blockers increase longevity in severe congestive cardiac failure
D. The one year mortality following clinical diagnosis is >60%
E. 20 -30% of deaths are due to arrhythmias

QUESTION 26

Acute respiratory distress syndrome (ARDS)

A. Does not occur in children
B. Affects the lung in a diffuse and homogenous manner
C. Cannot be diagnosed in the presence of severe left ventricular failure
D. Should be treated with corticosteroids in the early stages
E. Has a mortality of 20-30%

QUESTION 27

Systemic inflammatory response syndrome (SIRS)

A. Is initiated by infection in over 80% of cases
B. Is more commonly caused by gram negative than gram positive organisms
C. Cannot be diagnosed until a patient is hypotensive despite adequate fluid resuscitation
D. Has a mortality of 40-60%
E. Should be treated with monoclonal antibodies effective against endotoxin

QUESTION 28

Transoesophageal echocardiography

A. Is contraindicated in the presence of oesophageal varices
B. Is not as good at detecting venous air embolism as praecordial doppler
C. Cannot be used to assess ejection fraction
D. Uses sound waves
E. Can be used to detect ischaemia

QUESTION 29

Definite indications for the use of fresh frozen plasma (FFP) include

A. Acute disseminated intravascular coagulation (DIC)
B. Following the transfusion of 4 units of SAG-M blood
C. Cardiac bypass surgery
D. Thrombotic thrombocytopaenic purpura (TTP)
E. Plasma exchange procedures

QUESTION 30

The following are normal values

A. Pulmonary Artery Wedge Pressure (PAWP) = 8-12 mmHg
B. Stroke Volume (SV) = 0.6-1.3 l
C. Cardiac Index (CI) = 2.5-4 l/min
D. Pulmonary Vascular Resistance (Indexed) (PVRI) = 1750-2500 dyne.sec.cm^{-5}.m^{-2}
E. Mixed Venous Saturation (SvO$_2$) = 50%

QUESTION 31

At birth in the term neonate

A. The ductus arteriosum is completely closed

B. The foramen ovale functionally closes over a period of 3 days

C. Cardiac output is dependent upon heart rate

D. Pulmonary vascular resistance is reduced by breathing

E. A patent ductus arteriosum is important in complex congenital heart disease

QUESTION 32

The following drugs taken in overdose can increase core temperature in excess of 40 degrees centigrade

A. Aspirin

B. Phenobarbitone

C. Cocaine

D. Amitriptyline

E. Tranylcypromine

QUESTION 33

The following are true concerning endotracheal and endobronchial tubes

A. A Carlens tube has side by side lumens and is designed to enter the left main bronchus

B. The Robertshaw double lumen tube has the advantage of a relatively low resistance to breathing

C. Cole tubes are less likely to kink than other similar internal diameter neonatal tubes due to thicker walls

D. A Brompton tube is equiped with three cuffs

E. A Jackson-Rees paediatric tube has a suction port inbuilt

QUESTION 34

The following drugs are considered safe for use in MH-susceptible patients

A. Desflurane

B. Amide local anaesthetics

C. D-tubocurare

D. Digoxin

E. Decamethonium

QUESTION 35

Sources of error in pulse oximetry include

A. Vasoconstricted digits
B. The presence of foetal haemoglobin
C. Dark coloured nail varnish
D. Tricuspid incompetence
E. High ambient light intensity

QUESTION 36

Hepatic cirrhosis is associated with

A. Palmar erythema
B. Gonadal atrophy
C. Decreased plasma albumin
D. A poor prognosis when the liver edge is palpable
E. Wilson's disease

QUESTION 37

Causes of hypophosphataemia include

A. Alcohol withdrawal
B. Treatment with magnesium salts
C. Diabetic ketoacidosis
D. Primary hyperparathyroidism
E. Acromegaly

QUESTION 38

An Acute Pain Service

A. Should consist of a consultant anaesthetist with junior anaesthetic support
B. Intervention should be based on assessment and frequent re-assessment of the pain
C. Education of patients and staff is an important goal
D. Should be based on the use of drug and non-drug therapeutic strategies
E. Has no effect on duration of hospital stay

QUESTION 39

Concerning the pharmacology of local anaesthetic solutions

A. The aminoamides are highly bound to albumin
B. A lignocaine plasma level of 10 mcg/ml corresponds to the onset of convulsions
C. Etidocaine has a higher plasma clearance than prilocaine
D. Adding adrenaline to bupivacaine helps minimise its toxicity
E. Acidosis decreases the convulsive threshold associated with local anaesthetic toxicity

QUESTION 40

Guidelines for day case surgery recommend

A. Surgery lasting less than 30 minutes
B. Only ASA 1 patients being accepted
C. Exclusion of patients requiring pre-operative investigation
D. Patients under 1 year of age being excluded
E. Overnight abstinence from driving post-operatively

QUESTION 41

During neonatal resuscitation

A. Hypoglycaemia is common
B. Cardiac massage is only performed if the neonate is asystolic
C. Exposure of the chest and abdomen is important to assess circulation and colour
D. If IPPV is required then the initial inspiration should be short
E. Bicarbonate administration prevents intraventricular haemorrhage

QUESTION 42

Deviation of the trachea to the right occurs in

A. Right sided pneumothorax
B. Massive left sided empyema
C. Goitre
D. Right pneumonectomy
E. Right upper lobe pulmonary collapse

QUESTION 43

When treating a patient with cardiac failure

A. IV frusemide only exerts its beneficial effects by diuretic activity
B. ACE inhibitors are ineffective if plasma renin activity is normal
C. Gout may be precipitated by the use of bumetanide
D. Drug interaction with digoxin is possible due to its low level of protein binding
E. Phosphodiesterase inhibitors can safely be used in patients with mitral stenosis

QUESTION 44

Gastrointestinal motility is affected by

A. 5 HT antagonists
B. Metoclopramide
C. H_2 receptor blockers
D. Neostigmine
E. Opioids via the chemoreceptor trigger zone

QUESTION 45

Oxygen delivery (DO$_2$) is dependent on the following variables

A. Myocardial afterload
B. Oxygen saturation of mixed venous blood
C. Haemoglobin concentration
D. Body temperature
E. Arterial oxygen saturation

QUESTION 46

The recommended maximal safe doses of the following anaesthetic agents are

A. Cocaine: 5 mg/kg
B. Prilocaine: 8 mg/kg
C. Hyperbaric bupivacaine: 1.5 mg/kg
D. Amethocaine: 1.5 mg/kg
E. Lignocaine: 6 mg/kg

QUESTION 47

In Addisons disease

A. There is a female preponderance
B. There is hyperpigmentation of skin exposed to light
C. Hypokalaemia occurs
D. A patient may present in shock
E. Postural hypotension is a feature

QUESTION 48

In a patient presenting with adult community acquired pneumonia

A. Chest pain is uncommon
B. Rusty coloured sputum suggests that the causative organism is 'atypical'
C. Hyponatraemia suggests the causative organism is Legionella pneumophilia
D. Positive blood cultures occur in 25% of cases due to Streptococcus pneumoniae
E. Gram positive cocci in the sputum suggests that Steptococcus pneumoniae is the causative organism

QUESTION 49

In bowel obstruction

A. Diarrhoea may be present
B. Small bowel obstruction occurs more slowly compared to large bowel obstruction
C. Ileocaecal reflux occurs
D. There is haemoconcentration
E. Sodium picosulphate is contra-indicated

QUESTION 50

Nosocomial sinusitis in critically ill patients

A. Is easily diagnosed in most patients due to purulent nasal discharge
B. Does not lead to meningitis
C. Is often due to unusual nosocomial pathogens
D. Is diagnosed with more certainty on CT scan compared with plain sinus radiographs
E. Is more common if the trachea is intubated by the nasal route compared with the oral route.

QUESTION 51

A pleural effusion

A. Is dull to percussion
B. Gives rise to bronchial breathing
C. Is uncommonly found in heart failure
D. Can be found in nephrotic syndrome
E. When associated with pancreatitis has a high amylase content

QUESTION 52

Concerning achalasia of the cardia

A. Degeneration of Auerbach's plexus occurs
B. Increased oesophageal peristalsis occurs
C. It affects women more commonly than men
D. It is similar to Chaga's disease
E. Dysphagia is typically worse with solids

QUESTION 53

Concerning acute pancreatitis

A. Serum amylase is an indicator of severity
B. Persistent diabetes mellitus is a complication
C. It may cause hypercalcaemia
D. It may be caused by hypocalcaemia
E. It may be caused by hyperlipidaemia

QUESTION 54

Concerning hiatus hernia

A. Rolling hernias are more common than sliding
B. Incidence decreases with age
C. It may present with iron-deficient anaemia
D. Rolling hernias are more likely to strangulate
E. It is no longer treated surgically

QUESTION 55

Myasthenia gravis

A. Is characterised by improved strength as a sustained effort is made

B. Has a higher incidence in females

C. May be exacerbated by erythromycin

D. Is a contraindication to the performance of a percutaneous dilatational tracheostomy

E. Causing a myasthenic crisis should be treated with immediate thymectomy

QUESTION 56

The oculo-cardiac reflex

A. Occurs on traction of the medial rectus

B. Does not occur with retro-bulbar block

C. May be obtunded by local anaesthetic infiltration of ocular muscles

D. Is most active in the elderly

E. Precipitates non-sinus dysrhythmias

QUESTION 57

Amniotic fluid embolus

A. Occurs more commonly in multiparous women

B. Is universally fatal

C. May present with convulsions

D. Was the third leading cause of death in the 1996 maternal mortality report

E. Refractory hypoxaemia and pulmonary hypertension are the first presenting features

QUESTION 58

The following drugs may cause urinary retention

A. Clomipramine

B. Prazosin

C. Morphine

D. Propofol

E. Phenoxybenzamine

QUESTION 59

The following are true of neuromuscular blockade

A. A train of four ratio less than 1 in depolarising blockade

B. A train of four ratio equal to 1 in dual (phase II) blockade

C. No fade elicited on double burst stimulation for non depolarising blockade

D. Ability to cough is the most useful indicator of adequate neuromuscular function

E. Fade on tetanic contraction during depolarising blockade

QUESTION 60

When considering direct intra-arterial blood pressure measurement

A. In the under-damped system the signal falls slowly to the baseline with overshoot
B. Soft catheters are a cause of damping
C. Optimal damping can be assessed by flushing the system
D. The mean pressure recorded is less in an over-damped system compared to an under-damped one
E. Optimal damping occurs when there is no overshoot of the baseline

QUESTION 61

In the bulk production and storage of oxygen

A. A VIE for oxygen storage should stand on asphalt to prevent the build up of static electricity
B. In a VIE oxygen is stored at $-183°C$.
C. Oxygen can be produced in a concentrator by passing air over a hydrous silicate
D. Care is required in the storage of oxygen on-site because of its flammability
E. The output from an oxygen concentrator is of the same purity as that produced by distillation of air

QUESTION 62

Regarding oxygen consumption and delivery

A. Oxygen delivery is the product of arterial PO_2 and cardiac output
B. Oxygen consumption is independent of oxygen delivery
C. Oxygen consumption can be measured using a pulmonary artery flotation catheter
D. Acidosis improves tissue oxygen availiabilty
E. The rate of oxygen consumption varies with basal metabolic rate

QUESTION 63

Concerning thyroid cancer

A. Anaplastic carcinoma carries a poor prognosis
B. Medullary carcinoma is confined to young patients
C. Papillary carcinoma carries a relatively good prognosis
D. Follicular carcinoma spreads by blood to lung and bone
E. Medullary carcinoma can be familial

QUESTION 64

Concerning nephrotic syndrome

A. Venous thrombosis is a complication
B. Hypercholesterolaemia can occur
C. Patients have increased susceptibility to pneumococci
D. Treatment involves diuretic therapy
E. Management includes increasing the amount of salt intake

QUESTION 65

Concerning gallstones

A. 20% are radio-opaque
B. Cholesterol stones usually suggest hypercholesterolaemia
C. Pigment stones are the commonest
D. Incidence is increased in females
E. They are a frequent post-mortem finding

QUESTION 66

Factors affecting the delivered concentration of vapour from a vaporizer include

A. Volume of volatile used
B. Fresh gas flow
C. Pumping effect
D. Surface area of gas / liquid interface
E. Two Tec 5 vaporizers in series both switched on

QUESTION 67

Signs associated with traumatic aortic rupture are

A. Tracheal deviation to the left
B. Fractures of the upper three ribs
C. Racoon eyes
D. Elevated hemidiaphragm
E. Widened mediastinum, which is 90% specific for aortic injury

QUESTION 68

Concerning the use of non-steroidal anti-inflammatory drugs (NSAIDs)

A. Short term use (less than 7 days) does not cause gastric erosions
B. Drugs that selectively inhibit cyclo-oxygenase 1 should result in a reduced incidence of side effects
C. Rectal administration abolishes the risk of gastroduodenal injury
D. Prolongation of the bleeding time by aspirin reverses if the drug is stopped for 5 days
E. Combination with ACE inhibitors increases the risk of renal ischaemia

QUESTION 69

In the transfusion of blood components

A. The plasma K^+ of stored blood can be up to 30 mmol/l
B. Levels of coagulation factors V and VIII are still 50% normal at 7 days in stored blood
C. Red blood cell viability is 35 days as a SAG-M preparation
D. Red blood cell viability is defined as 50% survival 12 hours after transfusion
E. SAG-M blood has a haematocrit of approximately 0.45

QUESTION 70

Considering reflex responses and the cardiovascular system

A. Cushings reflex is a result of central nervous system ischaemia
B. The Bainbridge reflex results in bradycardia
C. Reflex tachycardia from systemic venous distension is abolished by vagotomy
D. Arterial baroreceptors respond equally to increases or decreases in blood pressure
E. Arterial baroreceptors provide chronic control of systemic blood pressure

QUESTION 71

Aldosterone secretion is decreased by

A. Conn's syndrome
B. Non-steroidal anti-inflammatory drugs (NSAID)
C. Renal artery stenosis
D. Heart failure
E. Hypoadrenalism

QUESTION 72

Evidence based medicine

A. Is the remit if the Cochrane group

B. Is an exercise in cost benefit analysis

C. Requires that all available literature on a subject is stratified into one of four groups

D. Will generate a number needed to treat

E. Is not necessary in anaesthetic practice

QUESTION 73

The following are associated with hypokalaemia

A. Diarrhoea

B. Salbutamol

C. Rhabdomyolysis

D. Paralytic ileus

E. Renal artery stenosis

QUESTION 74

Absolute indications for one lung anaesthesia include

A. Prevention of infection from the other lung

B. Oesophagogastrectomy

C. Right upper lobectomy

D. Isolation of pulmonary haemorrhage

E. Laser resection of bronchotracheal stenosis

QUESTION 75

Percutaneous dilatational tracheostomy

A. Is performed through the cricothyroid membrane

B. Results in a higher incidence of tracheal stenosis than surgical tracheostomy

C. Should be performed with the neck partially flexed to avoid damage to the upper pole of the thyroid gland

D. Should be performed in all patients requiring an artificial airway for greater than 1 week

E. Can cause a reduction in minute volume

QUESTION 76

Entonox

A. Is most commonly used in a size E cylinder
B. Should be stored in blue and white cylinders according to international standards
C. Should not be stored below 20°C
D. Cylinders should be rewarmed and rotated if separation of the component gases has occurred
E. An 'entonox valve' is a one stage valve used with a pin index system

QUESTION 77

Concerning transport of the critically ill

A. The patient should ideally lie parallel to the axis of acceleration
B. The patient must leave immediately for a neurosurgical facility once an intracranial haematoma has been diagnosed
C. Size E oxygen cylinders hold 340 litres when full
D. Aeromedical transfer should be the first choice if available
E. Measurement of heart rate by palpation is an acceptable alternative to ECG measurement

QUESTION 78

The following can mimic the chest pain of myocardial infarction

A. Pericarditis
B. Oesophageal rupture
C. Spontaneous pneumothorax
D. Thoracic aortic dissection
E. Pulmonary embolism

QUESTION 79

The femoral nerve

A. Arises from L1, L2 and L3
B. Passes under the inguinal ligament medial to the femoral artery
C. Supplies skin to the medial part of the thigh
D. Is damaged in fractures to the neck of the fibula
E. Gives rise to the saphenous nerve

QUESTION 80

Concerning nutritional support in the critically ill

A. Septic complications are 25% less frequent in patients given enteral rather than parenteral feeding

B. Elemental feeds stimulate pancreatic exocrine secretion less than complex feeds

C. The duration of a post operative ileus correlates with the degree of gut handling at surgery

D. The frequency of diarrhoea in patients receiving enteral nuitrition on the ICU is about 25%

E. Continuous enteral feeding leads to increased gram negative colonisation of the upper GI tract

QUESTION 81

In patients with renal dysfunction

A. Protein binding of basic drugs (pKa >7.4) is unaltered

B. Protein binding of drugs is affected by the degree of uraemia

C. The half life of drugs increases significantly below a creatinine clearance of 50 ml/min

D. Phenothiazines are safe to use as pre-medicants

E. Uraemia has no effect on hepatic drug metabolism

QUESTION 82

Concerning the brachial plexus

A. The trunks divide into anterior and posterior branches beneath the clavicle

B. It lies in the anterior triangle of the neck

C. The musculocutaneous nerve arises at the lower border of pectoralis minor

D. The median nerve is formed from the posterior cord

E. The circumflex nerve may be damaged in fractures to the neck of humerus

QUESTION 83

Concerning the diagnosis of brain stem death

A. Clinicians performing the tests should have been registered for 5 years

B. An isoelectric EEG excludes neurological recovery following cerebral ischaemia

C. The time of death is at the cessation of the heart beat or removal of the heart if the patient becomes a donor

D. The interval between the two set of tests should be in excess of 4 hours

E. The tests involve demonstrating brain stem areflexia with 5 tests and confirming persistent apnoea

QUESTION 84

Concerning the larynx

A. The recurrent laryngeal nerve supplies the mucous membrane above the vocal cords
B. The cricothyroid muscle is supplied the external laryngeal nerve
C. The vocal cords are lined by stratified squamous epithelium
D. It is raised by the infrahyoid muscle
E. The rima glottidis lies between the vocal folds

QUESTION 85

Concerning gas embolism

A. Neurosurgery performed in the sitting position carries a 25% incidence
B. A right lateral head down position is recommended
C. There is a sudden increase in lung dead space
D. The central venous pressure and end tidal CO_2 will fall
E. Doppler is the most sensitive means of detecting air

QUESTION 86

Concerning electroencephalogram (EEG) monitoring

A. The potentials recorded bear no relation to oxygen consumption
B. Alpha activity is those potentials with the highest frequency
C. Thiopentone infusion can cause 'burst suppression'
D. Thiopentone can cause loss of all electrical activity
E. The ECG can be derived from the EEG

QUESTION 87

Concerning paracetamol overdose

A. Induced liver enzymes offer some protection
B. Liver function tests are the best guide to severity
C. Treatment with N - acetyl cysteine offers protection up to 24 hours after ingestion
D. 10 grammes (20 tablets) is sufficient to cause liver necrosis
E. Abdominal pain is not a feature

QUESTION 88

The following correctly identify anatomical levels

A. Cricoid cartilage at the level of the second thoracic verebra

B. The body of the hyoid bone at the level of the fourth cervical vertebra

C. Upper border of thyroid cartilage at the level of the sixth cervical vertebra

D. The isthmus of the thyroid gland between the levels of the second to fourth tracheal rings

E. The thoracic termination of the trachea at the sixth thoracic vertebra

QUESTION 89

The following biochemical values will indicate that acute renal failure (ARF) is pre-renal in origin

A. 24 hour urinary volume 800 ml

B. Urine sodium concentration > 40 mmol / litre

C. Urine : serum urea concentration > 10 : 1

D. Urine : serum osmolality < 1.1 : 1

E. Serum creatinine 185 mmol / litre

QUESTION 90

Concerning the management of cardiogenic shock

A. The optimal left ventricular filling pressure is 12 mmHg

B. The use of dobutamine shows greater haemodynamic benefit than dopamine

C. Vasodilators tend to increase hypoxaemia

D. Salbutamol infusion can increase cardiac output without affecting pulmonary capillary wedge pressure (PCWP)

E. Catecholamine therapy decreases myocardial oxygen consumption

Exam 3: Answers

ANSWER 1

A. FALSE   B. FALSE   C. FALSE   D. TRUE   E. TRUE

Propofol, an alkyl phenol, is highly lipid soluble and has a volume of distribution at steady state of 400-700 litres. In the liver it is either conjugated to form propofol glucuronide or is metabolised to 2,6-disopyl 1,4-quinol and then conjugated. Less than 1% is excreted unchanged in the urine. It is licensed for use in combination with lignocaine (which reduces the 5-30% incidence of pain on injection) and alfentanil. It has, to date, been safely used in patients with porphyria.

Ref: Nimmo, Rowbotham and Smith. Anaesthesia (Second Edition) Blackwell Scientific Publications. Ch4.

ANSWER 2

A. FALSE   B. TRUE   C. TRUE   D. TRUE   E. FALSE

There are a wide variety of surface techniques and local nerve blocks to provide upper airway anaesthesia. The safe dose of cocaine topically is up to 3mg/kg but it must be remembered that the dose of different local anaesthetics must be considered cumulatively. Airway obstruction may follow glossopharyngeal nerve block due to relaxation of musculature around the base of the tongue. Superior laryngeal nerve block may be performed by local application of anaesthetic (piriform fossae), or by nerve block at the inferior surface of the greater cornu of the hyoid bone deep to the thyrohyoid membrane. Different sources describe injecting local anaesthesia at different stages of the respiratory cycle, one specific time is not a requirement.

Ref: Yentis, Hirsch & Smith. Anaesthesia A to Z. Intubation, awake.
Ref: Miller. Anesthesia. Airway management.

ANSWER 3

A. TRUE   B. TRUE   C. TRUE   D. FALSE   E. FALSE

The normal ICP is 0-10 mmHg and requires active treatment when it is 25-30 mmHg. A III nerve palsy and decerebrate rigidity are signs of tentorial herniation.

Ref: Miller. Anesthesia 3rd ed. pp1897

ANSWER 4

A. FALSE   B. TRUE   C. TRUE   D. TRUE   E. FALSE

The arterial pressure trace provides more information than the pressure values alone. The initial peak seen is due to the jet of blood from the left ventricle impacting on the slowly moving blood in the aorta. The shoulder is due to a volume displacement wave in the aorta. The down-slope of the trace from here represents the flow of blood into the peripheral circulation. This reflects the peripheral circulatory tone. A second hump may be then seen as the volume displacement wave is reflected. The dicrotic notch present in centrally measured pressure is not seen in the peripheral trace. A significant difference in the height of the initial peak and the subsequent volume displacement wave (shoulder) is seen in atherosclerosis, hypovolaemia with vasoconstriction, and inotropic therapy. Tracings from more peripheral arteries have increasing impedance as the vessels narrow. This increases the pressure wave amplitude so systolic pressures MEASURED in the dorsalis pedis may be 20 mmHg greater than that in the radial artery. The mean pressure measured anywhere within the system is, however, consistent with central mean pressure. Spontaneous ventilation causes a fall in pressure during inspiration and a rise during expiration due to changes in ventricular afterload and interdependence.

Ref: Kirkland, L.L. and Veremakis, C. (1993) Arterial Pressure Monitoring. In: Carlson, R.W. and Geheb, M.A. (Eds.) Principles and Practice of Medical Intensive Care, pp. 251-256. Philadelphia: W B Saunders

ANSWER   5
A. TRUE   B. FALSE   C. FALSE   D. TRUE   E. TRUE

In Mallampati's assessment class 1 allows uvula, faucial pillars and soft palate to be seen. In class 2 the uvula and soft palate will be seen while in class 3 only the soft palate is visible. No direct assessment of the vocal cords is made. The distance between hyoid and mandible should be at least 2 fingerbreadths and mouth opening should be at least a similar distance. The distance from the mandibular symphysis to the thyroid should be at least three fingerbreadths with the head extended. Patients with scleroderma may be difficult to intubate because of tight perioral skin or temporo–mandibular joint involvement. Airway management of the patient with sarcoidosis may be complicated by the presence of abnormal lymphoid tissue.

Ref: Craft & Upton. Key topics in anaesthesia. Intubation- difficult.
Ref: Miller Anesthesia. Chapter 42. Airway management

ANSWER   6
A. FALSE   B. FALSE   C. TRUE   D. TRUE   E. TRUE

Respiratory volumes (FRC, TLC, RV) are reduced in restrictive disease. FEV_1, FEV_1/FVC ratio and FEF25-75 are reduced in obstructive disease.The MMV is a measure of the maximum ventilatory volume in 1 minute. It measures similar functions to the FEV_1, but has been shown to be valuable in predicting post-operative course. In determining the feasibility of lung resection, a predicted post-operative FEV_1 of > 800 ml is acceptable for surgery. Closing capacity is a sensitive indicator of alterations in the uniformity of ventilation. This may be due to changes associated with smoking.

Ref: Frye, M.D. and Olsen, N. (1990) Respiratory Function Tests. In: Scurr, C., Feldman, S. and Soni, N. (Eds.) Scientific Foundations of Anaesthesia; The Basis of Intensive Care, 4th edn. pp. 279-286. Oxford: Heinemann Medical Books

ANSWER   7
A. TRUE   B. FALSE   C. TRUE   D. FALSE   E. TRUE

There are several types of intracranial pressure monitors. The extradural fibreoptic probe is laid between the dura and skull via a burr hole. It has low infection rates but CSF drainage is impossible and accuracy less reliable. A subarachnoid screw may also be applied via a burr hole. It is more accurate and capable of CSF drainage but infection rates are higher. A ventricular drain placed during craniotomy is highly accurate with easy CSF drainage possible but infection rates are highest. An intracerebral transducer placed within the brain tissue is also possible. The waveform produced resembles an arterial waveform corresponding to the pulsations of large vessels within the brain. The normal mean intracranial pressure is 7-15 mm Hg in the supine position. Active management is usually advocated at pressures over 15-30 mm Hg depending on the underlying condition.

Ref: Yentis, Hirsch, Smith. Anaesthesia A to Z. Butterworth Heinemann.

ANSWER 8

A. FALSE   B. FALSE   C. FALSE   D. TRUE   E. TRUE

The neuro-hormonal response to a major burn injury leads to marked hypermetabolism with a strong catabolic hormonal predominance. A patient's daily calorific needs can be estimated from the Curreri formula:-

Needs(kcal) = (25kcal/Kg body weight) + (40kcal/%burn)

Therefore this gentleman would require 2500 + 2000 = 4500 kcal / day

Due to the hypermetabolism the body thermostat is set 1-1.5 degrees above 37 therefore a temperature of 38-39 degrees centigrade is quite normal in the first week and in the absence of any other signs does not suggest infection. There is no place for the use of prophylactic antibiotics in the management of burn patients except as a single dose to cover peri-operative procedures. Burn patients, due to their hypermetabolic response, generate large amounts of CO_2 and normally increase their minute ventilation dramatically to maintain normocapnia. If adequate analgesia is utilised with opioids and/or there is any respiratory insult or impairment then hypercapnia will ensue and, if ventilated, to avoid excessive airway pressures permissive hypercapnia may need to be used. In the acute phase, i.e. until most of the oedema is reabsorbed, tracheostomies should be avoided. There have been reports of fatal dislocation of tracheostomy tubes therefore naso/orotracheal intubation is initially recommended. Tracheostomy should be considered after the acute phase as an elective procedure. As well as reducing postoperative catabolism enteral omega-3 fatty acids, arginine and nucleotides (RNA) appear to improve the immune response and there is also evidence that medium-chain-triglycerides may be more beneficial than long-chain-triglycerides.

Ref: Current Anaesthesia and Critical Care.1996; Vol 7, No 1:pg 31-36. Intensive care treatment of burn patients.

ANSWER 9

A. FALSE   B. FALSE   C. FALSE   D. TRUE   E. FALSE

Patients with a GCS of less than 9 have severe brain injury. Traumatic brain injury is ultimately responsible for death or long term disability in a majority of multiply injured patients. About 40% of patients with closed head injury ultimately die and 13% remain in a persistent vegetative state. Only about 20% of patients with head injury will be operated on immediately and clean steroid muscle relaxants are preferable to those that can release histamine which occasionally increases ICP. The normal ICP is 5-15 mm Hg. Artificial hyperventilation has been shown to be effective in reducing ICP but it may induce cerebral ischaemia through vasoconstriction, particularly if there is decreased cerebral blood flow.

Ref: Current Anaesthesia and Critical Care 1996; Vol 7, No 3: pg 125-138. Anaesthetic management of the trauma patient in the operating theatre.

ANSWER 10

A. FALSE   **B. FALSE**   **C. FALSE**   **D. FALSE**   **E. TRUE**

A precordial thump is only recommended for witnessed arrests where it may help in pulseless VT and in VF very early on in resuscitation. Many drugs can be given by the endotracheal tube but concentrated sodium bicarbonate and calcium salt solutions are too irritant. The dose of adrenaline for adults is 1mg (children should initially receive 10mcg/kg) and the intra-cardiac route is no longer recommended routinely. 'High-dose' adrenaline is not specifically recommended more for one age group or another but some literature at present would lean towards it having more of a role in paediatric resuscitation.

Ref. Craft & Upton. Key topics in Anaesthesia. Cardiopulmonary resuscitation.

ANSWER 11

A. FALSE   **B. TRUE**   **C. FALSE**   **D. FALSE**   **E. TRUE**

Mitral stenosis is usually the result of rheumatic fever with a distorted and partly fused valve secondarily calcifying. Slow deterioration with dyspnoea, pulmonary oedema, chest pain, palpitations and haemoptysis occurs. Left atrial pressure is chronically raised and pulmonary hypertension occurs. Atrial contraction will contribute 30% of ventricular filling and if atrio-ventricular pacing is needed a long P-R interval will help filling of the ventricle. Cardiac output will usually not be helped by afterload reduction in the setting of a normal blood pressure since the obstruction is at mitral valve level. Pulmonary vascular resistance is a serious problem with right ventricular failure being a risk. If pulmonary vascular resistance increases the right ventricle may further distend and the inter-ventricular septum intrude on left ventricular function. Due to the pulmonary hypertension the pulmonary diastolic pressure will often be considerably above the pulmonary wedge pressure.

Ref: Hensley The practice of cardiac anaesthesia. Little, Brown. Anaesthetic management for the treatment of valvular heart disease.

ANSWER 12

A. FALSE   **B. TRUE**   **C. TRUE**   **D. FALSE**   **E. TRUE**

Storage of arterial blood gases at room temperature allows continued metabolism of the leukocytes and this causes a fall in PO_2 and pH. Air bubbles within the sample will alter the PO_2 and cause a fall in PCO_2 as the gas diffuses into the bubbles. Excessive heparin remaining in the syringe will cause a fall in PCO_2 but the pH will remain constant. A fall in blood temperature leads to a fall in PO_2, PCO_2 and a rise in pH. So if the specimen were analysed at an inappropriately high temperature the PO_2 would be inaccurately high.

Ref: Urbina, L.R. and Kruse, J.A. (1993) Blood Gas Analysis and Related Techniques. In: Carlson, R.W. and Geheb, M.A. (Eds.) Principles and Practice of Medical Intensive Care, pp. 235-250. Philadelphia: W B Saunders

ANSWER 13

A. FALSE   **B. TRUE**   **C. TRUE**   **D. TRUE**   **E. TRUE**

The coordinated cardiovascular response to haemorrhage involves a range of neural and humoral pathways. There is tachycardia due to sympathetic nervous system stimulation however this is not part of the Bainbridge reflex which is a tachycardia due to atrial or systemic venous distension. As a part of the sympathetic nervous system drive, the adrenal medulla releases catecholamines including a predominant amount of noradrenaline. Renin released from the juxtaglomerular cells due to decreased renal artery pressure or decreased sodium delivery to the distal tubule causes conversion of angiotensinogen to angiotensin I. Angiotensin II and III release aldosterone. Vasopressin released from the posterior pituitary produces increased free water reabsorption. Atrial natriuretic peptide is synthesised and stored in human atrial myocytes and is released in response to increased vascular volume especially from the right atrium.

Ref: Prys-Roberts & Brown. International Practice of Anaesthesia. Chapter 22.

ANSWER 14

A. TRUE   B. FALSE   C. TRUE   D. TRUE   E. FALSE

Progressive hypertension and bradycardia (Cushing response) is a reponse to an acute rise in intracranial pressure. Subdural haematoma is much more common than extradural haematoma. Extradural haematoma is characterised by loss of consciousness followed by a return of consciousness (lucid interval) and then a further deterioration in consciousness and a contralateral hemiparesis. In basal skull fractures there maybe CSF otorrhoea, rhinorrhoea, mastoid ecchymosis (Battles sign), orbital ecchymosis (racoon eyes) and haemotympanum.

Not all depressed skull fractures require operation. Any fragment depressed more than the thickness of the skull may require elevation of the bony fragment.

Ref. Advanced Trauma Life Support Student Manual. American College of Surgeons.

ANSWER 15

A. TRUE   B. TRUE   C. FALSE   D. TRUE   E. FALSE

Indications for mechanical ventialtion are in the main relative. Along with measurable physio-logical parameters the cause of respiratory failure and pattern of breathing must be reviewed. The normal values used are a MV<6 >15 l/min, TV<5ml/kg or VC<15 ml kg, an A-a grad >300 mmHg, FEV1 < 45%of VC.

Ref: Nunn JF. Applied Respiratory Physiology. Butterworth.

ANSWER 16

A. TRUE   B. TRUE   C. TRUE   D. TRUE   E. FALSE

The wet spirometer (such as the Benedict-Roth) uses a liquid seal between static and moving parts to measure volumes. A Bourdon gauge is used to measure high pressures as well as temperature and flow. An aneroid gauge consists of metal bellows and is used to sense smaller pressures. They are used commonly to measure blood pressure or to monitor pressures developed by ventilators. Diaphragm gauges are how most physiological pressure measurements are now made by sensing the movement of a flexible diaphragm and converting this into electrical energy. The liquid manometer is the basis of measurement of pressure and depends upon the principle that the pressure exerted by a column of fluid equals the product of the height of the column, the density of the fluid and acceleration due to gravity.

Ref: Sykes, Vickers, Hull. Principles of Measurement and Monitoring in Anaesthesia and Intesive Care. 3rd Edition. Blackwell Scientific Publications.

ANSWER   17

A. TRUE   B. FALSE   C. TRUE   D. FALSE   E. FALSE

Treatment of acute myocardial infarction involves symptomatic relief then infarct modification.

Cardiac pain that is not relieved by sublingual or buccal nitrate requires opiate therapy. The resulting anxiolysis and vaso/veno-dilatation reduce cardiac work. Apart from thrombolytic therapy and aspirin the only other treatment consistently shown to improve outcome when administered acutely is intravenous beta-blockade. Early ACE-inhibitor treatment favourably alters left ventricular remodelling so reducing dilatation and improving outcome (GISSI 3, ISIS 4 & SMILE). Despite enthusiasm in the 1980's, ISIS 4 showed that magnesium had no benefit as a primary agent in acute MI. The latest study on calcium antagonists (SPRINT 2) showed that nifedipine started within 48 hours of an acute MI resulted in a higher mortality.

Ref: Postgrad Med Journal 1995; 71: 534-541. The management of acute myocardial infarction

ANSWER   18

A. TRUE   B. TRUE   C. FALSE   D. TRUE   E FALSE

This lesion involves 1/3000 live births. There are many variants but 90% of lesions involve oesophageal atresia with a fistula from trachea to distal oesophagus. Associated congenital anomalies are present in 50% of neonates and cardiac anomalies are present in 20-25%. A soft oesophageal tube should be passed prior to repair to help remove secretions. After intubation the bevel of the endotracheal tube should lie posteriorly to help avoid intubating the fistula and the repair should be performed prior to gastrostomy to prevent ventilation difficulties due to gas loss via a decompressed stomach.

Ref: Stehling L. Common problems in pediatric anesthesia. Chapter 6.

ANSWER   19

A. TRUE   B. FALSE   C. FALSE   D. TRUE   E. TRUE

Plasma glucose is normally maintained at 4-6 mmol/l. Glucose entry into cells is mainly allowed by the presence of insulin, however cerebral neurones are permeable to glucose at all times without the presence of insulin. Muscle cells are also able to take up glucose at times of maximal exercise without the presence of insulin. At glucose concentrations of >10 mmol/l glucose will be lost in the urine.

Ref: Guyton. Review of Medical Physiology. Insulin, Glucagon & Diabetes.
Ref: Yentis, Hirsch, Smith. Anaesthesia A to Z. Glucose, Glucagon. Glucose reagent sticks.

ANSWER   20

A. TRUE   B. TRUE   C. FALSE   D. TRUE   E. TRUE

Dystrophica myotonica is an autosomal dominant condition causing progressive muscle weakness, ptosis, thinning of facial muscles. Other features include a mild intellectual impairement and a low serum IgG.

Ref: Hirsch, Yentis & Smith. Anaesthesia A to Z. Butterworth Heineman. p149

ANSWER 21

A. TRUE   B. FALSE   C. TRUE   D. FALSE   E. FALSE

Myasthenia gravis is an autoimmune disease, resulting from the production of antibodies against the acetylcholine receptors of muscle endplates. Medical treatment is aimed at :-

- enhancing neuromuscular transmission with anticholinesterases
- suppressing the immune system by corticosteroids and azathioprine
- decreasing the circulating antibody level by plasmapheresis

Physostigmine is an anticholinesterase but is not used in myasthenia as it is not a quaternary compound and therefore crosses the blood brain barrier, having profound CNS effects. 3,4-diaminopyridine is used in the management of Eaton-Lambert syndrome. By increasing transmitter release it antagonises neuromuscular and autonomic system disorders.

Ref: Canadian Journal of Anaesthesia. 1992, Vol 39, No 5, pg 476 -486. Anaesthesia and Myasthenia Gravis

ANSWER 22

A. TRUE   B. TRUE   C. TRUE   D. TRUE   E. TRUE

Secondary analgesics are useful in specific painful conditions but otherwise do not possess intrinsic nonspecific analgesic activity.

Cyproheptadine and other 5-HT antagonists such as methysergide and pizotifen are useful in the management of migraine.

Calcitonin provides symptomatic relief in patients with Paget's disease.

Baclofen is a GABA antagonist and is useful in the management of the pain that arises due to spasm of striated muscle that may occur with upper motor neurone lesions and spasmodic torticollis.

Propranolol is occasionally used in the prophylaxis of migranous neuralgias and 'atypical' facial pain.

Carbamazepine is the drug of choice in trigeminal neuralgia.

Ref: Calvey and Williams. Principles and Practice of Pharmacology for Anaesthetists. Blackwell Scientific Publications. Ch10.

ANSWER 23

A. FALSE   B. TRUE   C. FALSE   D. FALSE   E. TRUE

The treatment of tetanus includes supportive care, heavy sedation, wound toilet, antibiotics and human tetanus immunoglobulin. The exotoxin responsible for the neurological manifestations travels mainly via motor neurones, and therefore plasmapheresis will be ineffective. It is useful in myasthenia gravis although this beneficial effect is only maintained for 4 to 7 days. It is therefore useful in managing a patient prior to thymectomy and in those suffering a myasthenic crisis. Botulism is treated by supportive measures, removal of unabsorbed toxin from the bowel (enemas), botulinus antitoxin and wound debridement (in the rare cases of wound botulism).

Salicylate overdose requires supportive care, reduction of further absorption (activated charcoal) and occasionally encouragement of an alkaline urine (not a forced diuresis). If severe acute or chronic overdose are present, haemodialysis is recommended. There is proven benefit of plasmapheresis in those with GBS and this should be undertaken at an early stage to gain the most benefit. There is also now increasing evidence of the benefit of administering human immunoglobulin, and it may be that both these therapies are equally efficacious.

Ref: Linton DM. Acute neurological disorders: perioperative and critical care management strategies. Current Anaesthesia and critical Care 1992;3:162-167.

ANSWER 24

A. TRUE   B. FALSE   C. FALSE   D. FALSE   E. TRUE

The A-delta fibres terminate mainly in lamina I of the dorsal horn from where second order neurones project in the contralateral spinothalamic tracts. The C fibres release glutamate and substance P principally in laminae II and III. The ascending slow pain pathways, after synapsing with interneurones in the substantia gelatinosa project widely in the brainstem, but only 10-20% pass directly to the thalalmus. The descending pathways release enkephalin and serotonin, the former having pre and post synaptic influences on incoming pain fibres.

Ref: Guyton and Hall. Textbook of Medical Physiology. Chapter 48. Somatic sensation.

ANSWER 25

A. FALSE   B. TRUE   C. FALSE   D. FALSE   E. FALSE

Once heart failure is clinically overt, the prognosis is poor with 1 year mortality in the range 34-58%; and arrhythmias account for 30-50% of deaths. ACE inhibitors are the only group of drugs shown to increase longevity in CCF. They block the renin-angiotensin system and reduce both preload and afterload; and cardiac output increases by 20%. Although useful in acute LVF, prolonged high dose diuretic therapy activates the renin-angiotensin and sympathetic systems, thus increasing cardiac afterload, reducing cardiac output and exacerbating the hyponatraemia, hypokalaemia and hypomagnesaemia.

Ref: T.E. OH. Intensive Care Manual. Butterworths. 3rd Ed. Ch 11. Heart failure

ANSWER 26

A. FALSE   B. FALSE   C. TRUE   D. FALSE   E. FALSE

ARDS was first described in 1967. One of the patients described was a child. Although 4 years later the same group reported on the adult respiratory distress syndrome, a recent consensus conference recommended a return to the original acute nomenclature. ARDS comprises hypoxia, radiographic changes and the absence of heart failure following exposure to one or more of many risk factors, both directly and indirectly to the lung. The damage results in an increased capillary permeability and the formation of low pressure pulmonary oedema. This causes V/Q mismatching and a reduction in compliance. Recent studies have demonstrated that some areas of the lung remain relatively unaffected, and others (usually the dependent areas) are severely affected. Treatment involves removing the underlying cause, careful fluid balance to avoid exacerbating the increases in lung water whilst maintaining adequate intravascular filling and tailoring ventilatory strategy to avoid ventilator induced lung injury whilst maintaining adequate respiratory function. Nitric oxide, high frequency ventilation, surfactant and extracorporeal lung assist may have a place but their role has yet to be defined. Steroids have no place in the acute phase, although case reports suggest they may alter the late, fibroproliferative phase. Mortality is >50%.

Ref: Beale R, Grover ER, Smithies M, Bihari D. Acute respiratory distress syndrome ("ARDS"): no more than a severe acute lung injury? British Medical Journal 1993;307:1335-1339

ANSWER 27

A. FALSE   B. TRUE   C. FALSE   D. TRUE   E. FALSE

SIRS is the response to a variety of clinical insults. Two or more of the following occur:

i)temperature >38°C or <36°C

ii)heart rate >90 beats/min

iii)respiratory rate >20 breaths/min or $PaCO_2$ <4.3 kPa

iv)WBC >12000/cubic mm or <4000/cubic mm, or >10% immature forms

The aetiology of SIRS includes trauma, thermal injuries, infections (responsible for approx. 50% of cases), aspiration, pancreatitis, multiple blood transfusions and pulmonary contusion. When infection is the cause, gram negative bacteria are identified in 50% of cases, and gram positive in 5-20%. Current opinion suggests that an uncontrolled immunoinflammatory response results in regional tissue hypoxia. Gastrointestinal injury (such as ischaemia/reperfusion) has been implicated by the translocation of bacteria or toxins into the portal circulation at a rate too high to be neutralised by the normal mechanisms. This has been convincingly proven in animals but not in humans. Interest in the use of anti-endotoxin monoclonal antibodies has waned following several large trials comparing their use in those with and without shock with placebos. The results indicated that following reliable diagnosis, there was no benefit with their use. Other cytokine antibodies are currently under investigation. Poor prognostic factors include inappropriate antibiotics, inadequate surgical treatment, chronic illness, gross physiological derangement and renal, hepatic or haematological failure on ICU admission.

Ref: Ahmed NA, Christou NV, Meakins JL. The systemic inflammatory response syndrome and the critically ill patient. Current Opinion in Critical Care 1995;1:290-305.

ANSWER 28

A. TRUE   B. FALSE   C. FALSE   D. TRUE   E. TRUE

Transoesophageal echocardiography uses sound waves to penetrate tissues. The amount of energy reflected back by tissues is dependent upon their density. Hence anatomical structures can be outlined by determining the "brightness" of the reflected energy and the time interval from transmission to reflection. It can be used to assess the ejection fraction, cardiac output, segmental wall ischaemia, valve function, aortic aneurysms and dissections as well as intracardiac air. It is more sensitive to air than doppler. Its use is contraindicated with oesophageal varices, strictures, oesophagitis and in those with previous oesophageal surgery.

Ref: Barash, Cullen, Stoelting. Clinical Anesthesia. J.B. Lippincott Company.

ANSWER 29

A. TRUE   B. FALSE   C. FALSE   D. TRUE   E. FALSE

Definite indications for use of FFP (British Committee for standards in Haematology):

Replacement of isolated factor deficiencies where specific or combined

Immediate reversal of warfarin effect

Acute DIC

Treatment of TTP

Conditional uses (in the presence of bleeding and disturbed coagulation) :

    Massive blood transfusion

Liver disease

Cardiopulmonary bypass surgery

Special paediatric indications

No justification for the use of FFP:

Hypovolaemia

Plasma exchange procedures

'Formula' replacement

Nuitritional support

Treatment of immunodeficiency states

Ref: Current Anaesthesia and Critical Care 1996; Vol 7, No 4: pg 192-196. The uses and limitations of blood and blood products in resuscitation and intensive care.

ANSWER 30

A. TRUE   B. FALSE   C. TRUE   D. FALSE   E. FALSE

Normal values should be known as they are easy fodder for multiple choice questions:

PAWP = 8-12 mmHg

MPAP = 9-16 mmHg

CVP = 0-8 mmHg

MAP = 65-100 mmHg

Cardiac Output (CO) = 4-8 l/min

CI = 2.5-4 l/min/m^2

SVRI = 1760-2600 dyne.sec.cm^{-5}.m^{-2}

PVRI = 44-225 dyne.sec.cm^{-5}.m^{-2}SvO$_2$ = 75%

SvO$_2$ = 75%

ANSWER 31

A. FALSE   B. FALSE   C. TRUE   D. TRUE   E. TRUE

The transitional circulation describes the circulation within the foetus. At birth this changes as a result of changes in systemic and pulmonary vascular resistance. Pulmonary vascular resistance falls with the first breath and removal of the lungs hypoxic enviroment. Systemic vascular resistance rises. Therefore the foramen ovale should snap shut and flow reverse in the PDA. The DA will functionally close over 2-3 days. Neonates are very dependent upon heart rate for their cardiac output, and in certain forms of complex congential heart disease a PDA is the only method of pulmonary blood flow.

Ref: Scurr, Feldman and Soni. Scientific Foundations 4th ed. Heinemann. pp 521.

ANSWER 32

A. TRUE   B. FALSE   C. TRUE   D. FALSE   E. TRUE

A core temperature > 40 degrees centigrade is a medical emergency requiring immediate intervention. Complications include coagulopathy, rhabdomyolysis, ATN, convulsion and cardiorespiratory depression. Salicylates uncouple oxidative phosphorylation. Amphetamines (including Ecstasy), monoamine oxidase inhibitors and cocaine are associated with hyperthermia. Hypothermia (<35 degrees centigrade) is usually due to CNS depressants, commonly alcohol, anti-depressants, phenothiazines and barbiturates. Rarely with the phenothiazines hyperthermia may occur as a result of the neuroleptic malignant syndrome.

Ref: BNF 1996; No 32: pg 18-26. Emergency treatment of poisoning. Current Anaesthesia and Critical Care 1996; Vol 7, No 2: pg 95-100. Concepts in the management of poisoning

ANSWER 33

A. FALSE   B. TRUE   C. TRUE   D. TRUE   E. TRUE

A Carlens tube is designed for the left main bronchus but has anterior-posterior lumens. The Robertshaw tube which can be left or right sided has side by side lumens and with rather wider lumens has a low resistance to gas flow. Cole tubes sometimes used for neonates have a shoulder which can cause irritation to the cricoid ring and are little used in anaesthesia. A Brompton tube has three lumens so that if the outer cuff for the bronchial lumen fails it has an inner replacement which will still function.

Ref: Yentis, Hirsch & Smith. Anaesthesia A to Z. Tracheal tubes & Endobronchial tubes
Ref: Ward. Anaesthetic equipment. Chapter 7. Breathing attachments and their components

ANSWER 34

A. FALSE   B. TRUE   C. FALSE   D. TRUE   E. FALSE

All potent volatile agents and the depolarizing muscle relaxants such as suxamethonium and decamethonium must be avoided in MH-susceptible individuals. D-tubocurare is considered unsafe as it has some depolarizing activity, the rest of the non-depolarizing relaxants are considered safe. In the past amide local anaesthetics were considered unsafe as in vitro they increased calcium efflux from the sarcoplasmic reticulum. However these effects required concentrations far in excess of plasma values achieved in clinical practice and are now considered safe along with the esters.

Ref: Miller. Anesthesia. Churchill Livingstone. 4th Ed, Ch31

ANSWER 35

A. TRUE   B. FALSE   C. TRUE   D. TRUE   E. TRUE

The a.c. signal sensed by a pulse oximeter is about 1-5% of the d.c. signal when the pulse volume is normal so this explains why they become inaccurate when the patient is vasoconstricted from the cold or hypovolaemia. Other sources of inaccuracy include nail varnish, large venous pulsations, as in tricuspid incompetence, and a high ambient light intensity or infrared heaters or diathermy. Foetal haemoglobin has very similar absorption characteristics to adult haemoglobin and therefore does not cause error.

Ref: Sykes, Vickers, Hull. Principles of Measurement and Monitoring in Anasethesia and Intensive Care. 3rd Edition. Blackwell Scientific Publications.

ANSWER 36

A. TRUE   B. TRUE   C. TRUE   D. FALSE   E. TRUE

The liver is responsible for the catabolism of oestrogen, growth hormone, glucocorticoids, insulin, glucagon and parathyroid hormone. It also synthesises plasma proteins and albumin. As such, loss of liver function in advanced cirrhosis leads to gonadal atrophy. Palmar erythema is a non-specific reddening of the palms which indicates a hyperdynamic circulation and is usually found in chronic liver disease. Other clinical features include spider naevi, caput medussae, ascites and liver flap. A serum albumin less than 25g/l is a poor prognostic indicator. Among the rarer causes of cirrhosis is an autosomal recessive condition of copper metabolism (Wilsons disease) in which copper can be deposited in the liver. This is treated with penicillamine which chelates copper.

Ref: Kumar & Clark. Clinical Medicine. Balliere Tindall. Chapter 5

ANSWER 37

A. TRUE   B. TRUE   C. TRUE   D. TRUE   E. FALSE

Alcohol withdrawal is a rare cause of hypophosphataemia and is due to a decreased phosphate intake, magnesium deficiency and, when it occurs, ketoacidosis. In diabetic ketoacidosis, hypophosphatamia is seen during the recovery phase when there is increased uptake of phosphate into depleted tissues. Magnesium and aluminium salts can bind phosphate, lowering serum levels. Parathyroid hormone is phosphaturic, so even though parathyroid hormone leads to an increased uptake of phosphate (and calcium) from the gut, the phosphate is excreted. Acromegaly causes hyperphosphataemia.

Ref: Marshall. Clinical Chemistry. Lippincott Company. Ch 14

ANSWER 38

A. FALSE   B. TRUE   C. TRUE   D. TRUE   E. FALSE

Successful management of acute pain has been shown to reduce mortality and morbidity, as well as reduced hospital stay and improved patient satisfaction. The Service should comprise a multi-disciplinary team including staff from all branches of the health care staff. Treatment should be planned pro-actively on an individual basis, and this is based on assessment and frequent re-assessment of the pain. Both drug and non-drug therapies should be used. The team should have a recognisable structure with clear lines of responsibility. Apart from directly treating the patient's pain the team should also be responsible for teaching patients and staff in pain management.

Ref: Cousins, M. (1994) Acute and post-operative pain. In: Wall, P.D. and Melzack, R. (Eds.) Textbook of Pain, 3rd edn. pp. 357-386. Edinburgh: Churchill Livingstone

ANSWER 39

A. FALSE   B. TRUE   C. FALSE   D. FALSE   E. TRUE

The aminoamides are highly protein bound, mainly to alpha acid glycoprotein and to a lesser extent albumin. Metabolic clearance is virtually equivalent to hepatic clearance and are in the following order bupivacaine < mepivacaine < lignocaine < etidocaine < prilocaine. There seems to be no clear relationship in this to either potency, lipid solubility or protein binding.

The plasma level at which different toxic effects occur with lignocaine are:-

PLASMA CONC. (mcg/ml)	SYMPTOMS
30	cardiovascular collapse
20	respiratory arrest
15	loss of consciousness

10	convulsions
6	minor CNS symptoms - visual/circumoral/drowsy
1	antiarrhythmic effect

Acidosis, either respiratory or metabolic, decreases the convulsive threshold increasing the chance of developing CNS toxicity and also prolongs the toxicity. The practice of adding adrenaline to bupivacaine in order to minimise the plasma levels is unwise as adrenaline enhances the toxicity of bupivacaine.

Ref: Current Anaesthesia and Critical Care. Churchill Livingstone. 1995. Vol 6, No 1, pg 41 - 47. The pharmacology of local anaesthetic drugs.

ANSWER 40
A. FALSE   B. FALSE   C. FALSE   D. FALSE   E FALSE

Day case surgery is surgery in which the patient both presents to hospital and returns home on the day of the procedure. It is recommended for surgery that is predicted to last less than one hour. Generally it should be confined to ASA 1 or 2 patients but ASA 3 patients are occasionally accepted. Patients may be screened in pre-operative clinics prior to admission and if necessary any investigations ordered. Age limits are controversial and vary between units. The usual lower age limit is < 6 months. Prior to discharge patients are told to abstain from alcohol, driving and operating machinery etc. for at least 24 hours.

Ref: Craft & Upton. Key Topics in Anaesthesia. Bios Scientific Publishers.

ANSWER 41
A. TRUE   B. FALSE   C. FALSE   D. FALSE   E FALSE

Neonatal resuscitation follows the principles of adult resus but the neonate must be dried and kept warm as a matter of priority. Gentle suction or tactile stimulation often provokes activity. If IPPV is necessary then the first inspiration should be 3- 5 secs to aid lung expansion. Bicarbonate should be diluted as the osmotic load can cause intracerebral haemorrhage.

Ref: Yentis, Hirsch, and Smith. Anaesthesia A-Z. Butterworths. pp 86

ANSWER 42
A. FALSE   B. TRUE   C. TRUE   D. FALSE   E. TRUE

The trachea is pushed away from the pneumothorax. Empyema is the presence of pus in the pleural cavity usually due to rupture of a lung abscess or secondary to pneumonia. If this causes bronchial collapse, the trachea maybe pulled towards the lesion. Goitre may lead to stridor and / or difficult intubation. Over several weeks pneumonectomy spaces fill with fluid and generalised fibrosis occurs. This causes no mediastinal or tracheal shift.

Ref: Mason & Swash. Hutchinson's Clinical Methods. Balliere Tindall. 8th edition. Chapter 8.

ANSWER 43
A. FALSE   B. FALSE   C. TRUE   D. FALSE   E. FALSE

Frusemide, given intravenously, relieves pulmonary oedema by arteriolar vasodilatation. This is independent of its diuretic actions. ACE inhibitors produce lowering of systemic vascular resistance and venous pressure, and reduce circulating catecholamines. This effect is independent of their ACE inhibition as they are effective if plasma renin activity is normal. Loop diuretics can cause hyperuricaemia as can thiazides. Digoxin is highly protein bound. This makes it liable to displacement (and consequent toxicity) by other drugs. Phosphodiesterase inhibitors are inodilating drugs and therefore may cause cardiovascular collapse in those with a fixed cardiac output.

Ref: Kumar and Clark. Clinical Medicine (Third Edition) Bailliere Tindall. Ch 11

ANSWER   44

A. FALSE   B. TRUE   C. FALSE   D. TRUE   E. FALSE

Ondansetron (5 HT antagonist) reduces nausea and vomiting by central activity. Opioids and metoclopramide have both central and local actions on gut motility. Neostigmine causes a rise in acetylcholine levels and will increase segmental contractions within the bowel.

Ref: Harrison, Healy and Thornton. Aids to Anaesthesia. Churchill Livingstone. pp 187

ANSWER   45

A. TRUE   B. FALSE   C. TRUE   D. TRUE   E. TRUE

DO_2 is estimated by multiplying the cardiac output and the oxygen content of arterial blood. Cardiac output is dependent on heart rate, preload, contractility and afterload and alterations in these will increase or decrease the output. Arterial oxygen content is estimated by multiplying the haemoglobin concentration, arterial oxygen saturation and 1.34 (each g of haemoglobin carries 1.34 ml of oxygen when 100% saturated). In addition, a tiny amount of oxygen is delivered dissolved in the blood which is equal to 0.003 multiplied by the PaO_2 in mmHg (0.0225 x PaO_2 in kPa). At a steady PaO_2, body temperature directly affects the oxyhaemoglobin dissociation curve, hypothermia shifting the curve to the left, resulting in a higher SaO_2. Mixed venous oxygen saturation is useful to calculate the oxygen content of mixed venous blood (in a manner analogous to the arterial oxygen content). Subtracting this from the arterial oxygen content and multiplying the result by the cardiac output gives the oxygen consumption (VO_2).

Ref: West. Respiratory Physiology- the essentials (4th Edition). Williams and Wilkins. Ch 6. Hillman and Bishop. Clinical Intensive Care. Cambridge University Press. Ch 17.

ANSWER   46

A. FALSE   B. TRUE   C. FALSE   D. TRUE   E. TRUE

"Safe" doses of local anaesthetic agents vary according to the state of health of the patient, the blood supply of the area they are administered to, and the concomitant use of vasoconstrictors. Nevertheless, this dose of cocaine is in excess of the commonly quoted maximum dose of 1.5 mg/kg, and most would accept that bupivacaine can be safely given in doses up to 2 mg/kg.

Ref: Yentis, Hirsch, Smith. Anaesthesia A-Z. Butterworths. pp 277

ANSWER   47

A. FALSE   B. TRUE   C. FALSE   D. TRUE   E. TRUE

The sex distrubution is equal and it can occur at any age. Hyperpigmentation of skin exposed to light, friction or pressure can occur. Gingival, scar, nipple, freckle, tongue or genital pigmentation can also occur secondary to the combined effects of beta lipotrophin and melanocyte stimulating hormone. Hyperkalaemia and hyponatraemia occur and this may cause an ascending neuromyopathy. An acute adrenal insufficiency ("Addisonian crisis") may lead on from chronic hypoadrenalism when there is not enough hormone reserve to meet the stress of trauma, infection or surgery. Postural hypotension results from a decreased circulating blood volume and dehydration.

Ref: Oh. Intensive Care Manual. 3rd edition. Butterworths. Part VI.

ANSWER   48

A. FALSE   B. FALSE   C. TRUE   D. TRUE   E. TRUE

The major presenting features of community acquired pneumonia are cough, fever and chest pain. Common causative organisms are Streptococcus pneumoniae, 'atypical' agents (Mycoplasma pneumoniae, Legionella pneumophila, Coxiella burnetti, Chlamydia psittaci and Chlamydia pneumoniae), Staphylococcus aureus and Haemophilus influenzae. Pneumococcal pneumonia is suggested by a sudden onset with rigors, early cough that produces rust coloured sputum, pleuritic chest pain, neutrophilia, well defined CXR changes and G$^+$ cocci in the sputum. Atypical pneumonia is more likely if the onset is gradual following a prodromal influenza like illness with the late appearance of a cough that becomes mucopurulent, patchy CXR changes and a poor response to penicillin. Hyponatraemia is a marker for Legionella pneumophila. Streptococcus pneumoniae infection should be treated with penicillin or cefotaxime ± vancomycin in cases of penicillin resistance. Atypical pneumonia should be treated with a macrolide (erythromycin/clarithromycin) with rifampicin or ciprofloxacin added for severe Legionella infection.

Ref: Mandal, Wilkins, Dunbar and Mayon-White. Lecture notes on infectious diseases (Fifth Edition). Blackwell Science. Ch 7.

ANSWER   49

A. TRUE   B. FALSE   C. TRUE   D. TRUE   E. TRUE

Diarrhoea may result from impaired intestinal absorption of water and electrolytes caused by progressive oedema of the bowel wall. Small bowel obstruction develops more quickly than large bowel obstruction largely due to reflux of large bowel contents through the ileo-caecal valve. Loss of fluid absorption from the gut leads to dehydration and associated haemoconcentration. Stimulant laxatives such as sodium picosulphate are contraindicated in bowel obstruction.

Ref: Barash, Cullen & Stoelting. Clinical Anaesthesia. J.B. Lippincott Company.

ANSWER   50

A. FALSE   B. FALSE   C. FALSE   D. TRUE   E. TRUE

Nosocomial sinusitis is under diagnosed in the ICU. It should be suspected in intubated ICU patients who have purulent nasal discharge (which is a minority of all those with the infection), those whose fever remains undiagnosed, or those who develop a fever whilst on 'appropriate' antibiotics. The incidence is higher in those with nasal tubes present, although the presence of infection in those with oral tubes suggests that poor sinus ventilation may play a role.

It may be complicated by bacteraemia, pneumonia, meningitis (especially in those with basal skull fractures), epidural abscess, subdural empyema, venous sinus thrombosis, brain abscess and orbital infections. Nosocomial sinusitis is commonly caused by Staph. aureus, Ps. aeruginosa, Gram -ve bacilli and other usual nosocomial pathogens. Polymicrobial infections are common. Diagnosis is best achieved using CT scanning and aspiration of the maxillary antrum (which is involved in 85% of cases). Five different radiographic views of the sinuses are required to make an accurate diagnosis – this is often impractical. Treatment is controversial but often entails removal of nasal tubes, topical decongestants/vasoconstrictors and antimicrobial therapy. Sinus drainage can then be performed if this therapy fails.

Ref: Mayhall CG. Nosocomial sinusitis in the intensive care unit. Current Opinion in Critical Care. 1996;2:366-370

ANSWER   51

A. TRUE   B. TRUE   C. FALSE   D. TRUE   E. TRUE

Pleural effusions are "stony" dull to percussion over the effusion. However, there is nearly always compressed and solid lung over their upper border, giving an area of bronchial breathing. Pleural effusions occur commonly in heart failure and nephrotic syndrome.

Ref: Weatherall, Ledingham & Warrell. Oxford Textbook of Medicine. 2nd edition. vol 2 section 15

ANSWER   52

A. TRUE   B. FALSE   C. FALSE   D. TRUE   E. FALSE

Achalasia is a disease of unknown cause affecting men and women equally between 30 and 60 years and occuring in ~1/100000 of the population per annum. It presents with dysphagia (which may be worse with liquids) and retrosternal pain. This is caused by absence of oesophageal peristalsis and failure of the lower oesophageal sphincter to relax. The tropical disease Chaga's caused by Trypanosoma cruzi produces identical changes. Patients are often malnourished and have recurrent pneumonia secondary to aspiration. The treatment of choice is Heller's procedure which is analogous to Ramsted's for pyloric stenosis.

Ref: McLatchie. Oxford Handbook of Clinical Surgery. Oxford University Press.

ANSWER   53

A. FALSE   B. TRUE   C. FALSE   D. FALSE   E. TRUE

Acute pancreatitis is associated with gallstones, possibly alcohol, and a number of rarer causes including viral infection, ischaemia, hyperparathyroidism (hypercalcaemia), hyperlipidaemia, hypothermia and drugs (eg. steroids and azathioprine). Serum amylase is usually high but does not reflect the severity of the disease. Hypocalcaemia occurs secondary to calcium sequestration in areas of fat necrosis. Persistent diabetes mellitus can occur if there is destrucion of a major part of the gland.

Ref: Yentis Hirsch and Smith. Anaesthesia A to Z. Butterworth Heinemann.

ANSWER 54

A. FALSE B. FALSE C. TRUE D. TRUE E. FALSE

Hiatus hernia is protrusion of the stomach through the diaphragmatic crura into the thorax. It is most commonly sliding (or type I) when the oesophago-cardiac junction and upper stomach move into the thorax, or rolling (type II) when the oesophago-cardiac junction remains intra-abdominal but part of the gastric fundus herniates. Rolling hernias are more likely to strangulate. Hiatus hernia is more common in the elderly, smokers and the obese. It causes epigastric pain, regurgitation and GI bleeding hence patients can present with iron-deficient anaemia. It is managed medically initially (H_2 receptor antagonists, weight loss and cessation of smoking) but large hernias unresponsive to medical therapy may require surgery.

Ref: Yentis Hirsch and Smith. Anaesthesia A to Z. Butterworth Heinemann.

ANSWER 55

A. FALSE B. TRUE C. FALSE D. FALSE E. FALSE

Myasthenia gravis is an autoimmune disease due to skeletal muscle acetyl choline receptor antibodies. It is characterised by weakness or exaggerated fatigue on sustained effort. It is rare in the first 2 years of life and affects twice as many females as males. 75% have thymic histological abnormalities. Ptosis and diplopia are the commonest presenting symptoms, but bulbar and limb weakness are also fairly common. Treatment includes anticholinesterase drugs (e.g. pyridostigmine), corticosteroids, immunosuppressants (eg. azathioprine and cyclophosphamide), thymectomy (which should be considered electively in any patient) and plasmapharesis. An acute deterioration may be due to infection, pregnancy or drugs including aminoglycosides, tetracyclines, local anaesthetics, muscle relaxants or analgesics. ICU admission must be strongly considered as the risks of aspiration, pneumonia and respiratory failure are high. The patient may require an increase in their anticholinesterase if a myasthenic crisis is present, or a decrease if a cholinergic crisis is present. The latter is suggested by diarrhoea, abdominal cramps, salivation, bradycardia and deterioration during an edrophonium challenge ('Tensilon test'). Intubation, ventilation, physiotherapy, nutrition, electrolyte supplementation and plasmapharesis/corticosteroids should be considered. Some patients may benefit from a tracheostomy to aid weaning and allow pulmonary toilet.

Ref: Oh. Intensive Care Manual. Butterworths. Ch 44.

ANSWER 56

A. TRUE B. FALSE C. TRUE D. FALSE E. TRUE

The oculo-cardiac reflex is bradycardia following traction on the extraocular muscles especially the medial rectus. Although bradycardia is the commonest arrhythmia, ventricular ectopics or a nodal rhythm can also occur. It is most active in children. Retrobulbar block does not reliably obtund the reflex whereas local anaesthetic infiltration around the muscles does.

Ref: Yentis Hirsch and Smith. Anaesthesia A to Z. Butterworth Heinemann.

ANSWER 57

A. TRUE B. FALSE C. TRUE D. FALSE E. TRUE

Amniotic fluid embolus occurs more commonly in multips and forced labour. It carries an 80% mortality but is rare.

Ref: Yentis, Hirsch and Smith. Anaesthesia A-Z. Butterworths. pp17

ANSWER   58

A. TRUE   B. FALSE   C. TRUE   D. FALSE   E. FALSE

All of the tricyclic and related drugs can cause urinary retention due to their antimuscarinic effects. Alpha adrenergic antagonists such as prazosin relax smooth muscle and may improve obstructive symptoms in benign prostatic hyperplasia. They may, however, cause urinary frequency and incontinence. Phenoxybenzamine does not share these effects. In the renal tract morphine may cause ureteric spasm and difficulty in micturating. Apart from several cases of discolouration of the urine following prolonged administration, propofol has no effects on the renal tract.

Ref: British National Formulary. 1996;32

ANSWER   59

A. FALSE   B. FALSE   C. FALSE   D. FALSE   E FALSE

The train of four (TOF) ratio is force of the fourth twitch divided by the force of the first. In depolarising blockade there are equal but reduced twitches in response to TOF therefore the ratio is 1. In non depolarising blockade the TOF is less than 1. A dual (phase II) blockade occurs when large amounts of suxamethonium are used and the depolarising block is gradually replaced by a non depolarising one with all the neuromuscular qualities of one. Double burst stimulation is used to assess recovery from non depolarising blockade. Two short tetanic stimulations eg 50 Hz for 60 mS are applied 750 mS apart. The second response is weaker than the first in non depolarising blockade. It is more sensitive at detecting fade than TOF. Fade is the gradual decrease in strength of muscle contraction during tetanic stimulation exaggerated in non depolarising blockade. It is thought to be caused partly by inadequate mobilisation of acetylcholine in presynaptic nerve endings at the neuromuscular junction compared with the rate of release. It is not present in depolarising muscle blockade.

Ref: Yentis, Hirsch, Smith. Anaesthesia A to Z. Butterworth Heinemann.

ANSWER   60

A. FALSE   B. TRUE   C. TRUE   D. FALSE   E. FALSE

Damping is the progressive diminution of oscillations in a resonant system caused by dissipation of stored energy. In an under-damped system (resonant) the recorded signal falls rapidly, overshoots the baseline and is then followed by a series of oscillations of decreasing amplitude. In an over-damped one it falls slowly and takes some time to reach the baseline but there is no overshoot. Optimal damping is a compromise between speed of response and accuracy of registration of amplitude of the pressure trace. It occurs when the overshoot to a signal is 7% of the original deflection and the speed of response is only slightly reduced. It is demonstrated when there is 1 undershoot followed by a small overshoot in response to a flush. Critical damping occurs when the signal falls rapidly with no overshoot. Mean pressures recorded in over-damped, under-damped and correctly damped systems are the same. Causes of over-damping include air bubbles or clots in the system and the use of soft walled catheters which distend in response to a pulse wave.

Ref: Sykes, Vickers, Hull. Priciples of Measurement and Monitoring in Anaesthesia and Intensive Care. 3rd Edition. Blackwell Scientific Publications.

ANSWER   61

A. FALSE   B. TRUE   C. TRUE   D. FALSE   E. FALSE

A vacuum insulated evaporator should be supported on concrete rather than asphalt since the latter is combustible. In a vacuum insulated evaporator oxygen is stored at -183°C. Care is required in on-site storage of oxygen but this is because it supports combustion, it is not flammable in itself. Oxygen can be produced by use of a concentrator where air is passed over a silicate called zeolite. The purity of oxygen from a concentrator is greater than 92% but not of the same purity as oxygen from the distillation of air which is 99.6% pure.

Ref: Craft & Upton. Key topics in anaesthesia. Oxygen.
Ref: Ward. Anaesthetic equipment. Chapter 4. Piped medical gases and vacuum systems.

ANSWER   62

A. FALSE   B. FALSE   C. TRUE   D. TRUE   E. TRUE

Oxygen delivery is the product of arterial oxygen content and cardiac output. In healthy people the rate of oxygen consumption is dependent upon metabolic rate and is independent of oxygen delivery above about 400 ml/min. This may be vey different in critically ill patients where pathological flow dependency has been suggested. Acidosis that may occur with falls in oxygen delivery below a critical level further improves oxygen unloading by altering the P50.

Ref:Scurr, Feldman and Soni. Scientific Foundations of Anaesthesia 4th ed. Ch 24 pp287

ANSWER   63

A. TRUE   B. FALSE   C. TRUE   D. TRUE   E. TRUE

Most cancers of the thyroid are primary carcinomas, though metastases do occur. Medullary carcinoma affects a wide age range of patients, carries a variable prognosis, and can be familial. Papillary carcinoma affects patients less than 30 years of age and carries a relatively good prognosis. Follicular carcinomas do metastasise to lung and bone, but the metastases are often susceptible to radioactive iodine treatment. Anaplastic carcinoma usually arises in the elderly and the prognosis is poor.

Ref: McLatchie. Oxford Handbook of Clinical Surgery. Oxford University Press.

ANSWER   64

A. TRUE   B. TRUE   C. TRUE   D. TRUE   E. FALSE

Nephrotic syndrome comprises proteinuria, oedema, hypercholesterolaemia and clotting disorders. About half the cases have hypercholesterolaemia and the rise in cholesterol is proportional to the fall in serum albumin. Arterial and venous thromboses can occur. The aetiology is multifactorial. There is an increase in fibrinogen and factor VIII while antithrombin III is lost in urine. Haemoconcentration and immobility also play a part. A low IgG level may be responsible for the increased susceptibility to pneumococci and other encapsulated organisms. Frusemide alone or with amiloride, to prevent potassium loss, are commonly used in varying doses depending on the degree of oedema. In nephrotic syndrome there is retention of salt and water within the interstitial space, this is due to renal hypoperfusion and an increase in aldosterone. Hence salt intake should be lowered.

Ref: Weatherall, Ledingham & Warrell. Oxford Textbook of medicine. 2nd edition section 18

ANSWER 65

A. FALSE   B. FALSE   C. FALSE   D. TRUE   E. TRUE

Gallstones are common in developed countries, affecting 10% over the age of 50. They are often silent and are a frequent post-mortem finding. 10% are radio-opaque. The majority of stones are mixed, with pure cholesterol stones commoner than pigment stones. Cholesterol stones rarely reflect hypercholesterolaemia. The incidence of gallstones increases with age and biliary stasis. They are more common in women.

Ref: McLatchie. Oxford Handbook of Clinical Surgery. Oxford University Press.

ANSWER 66

A. FALSE   B. TRUE   C. TRUE   D. TRUE   E. FALSE

Factors affecting the delivered concentration of vapour include the splitting ratio, the saturated vapour pressure of the agent, the temperature of the liquid and the surface area of the gas / liquid interface. The fresh gas flow can affect the output of older vaporizers. Tec 5 vaporizers in series cannot be switched on concurrently. The surface area for vaporization of the volatile agent may be increased with the use of wicks and baffles (plenum vaporizer), the use of a cowl to direct the fresh gas flow onto / into the liquid (Boyles bottle) or by the production of many tiny bubbles with a sintered brass or glass diffuser (copper kettle vaporizer).

Ref: Yentis, Hirsch, Smith. Anaesthesia A to Z. Butterworth Heinemann.

ANSWER 67

A. FALSE   B. TRUE   C. FALSE   D. FALSE   E. FALSE

The thoracic aorta is at risk in any decelerating traumatic injury and a widened mediastinum may be overlooked on a supine CXR. This is a sensitive sign of aortic rupture, but is not very specific as 90% of widened mediastinums are due to venous bleeding. Signs associated with aortic rupture are:- Wide mediastinum, Pleural capping, Left haemothorax, Tracheal deviation to the right, Depression of the left mainstem bronchus, Loss of the aortic knob, Deviation of the nasogastric tube to the right, Fracture of the upper three ribs, Fracture of the thoracic spine. Racoon eyes are associated with base of skull fractures and an elevated hemidiaphragm is associated with diaphragmatic rupture.

Ref: Current Anaesthesia and Critical Care. 1996; Vol 7, No 3: pg 139-145 Care of trauma patients in the intensive care unit

ANSWER 68

A. FALSE   B. FALSE   C. FALSE   D. FALSE   E. TRUE

The effects of NSAIDs are due to their ability to inhibit cyclo-oxygenase. At least two isoenzymes are present. Cyclo-oxygenase 1 is responsible for homeostasis of renal blood flow, gastric cytoprotection and endothelial anti-thrombogenicity, and inhibition of this isoenzyme leads to side-effects. Cyclo-oxygenase 2 promotes the facilitation of pain and inflammation. Known risk factors for renal ischaemia occurring following the administration of NSAIDs are advanced age, hypovolaemia, hypotension, cardiac failure, hepatic cirrhosis and the combination with ACE inhibitors. Aspirin irreversibly inhibits platelet cyclo-oxygenase leading to reduced thromboxane A2 production and prolongation of the bleeding time. This anti-haemostatic effect is reversed as new platelets are formed, but may last for up to 15 days. Endoscopic evidence of erosions is evident in almost all subjects following NSAIDs administration as early as 24 hrs. However, their is little evidence to assess the risk of short term use causing clinically relevant ulceration. Injury is caused by both local and systemic routes, and therefore rectal administration reduces the risk but does not abolish it.

Ref: Halliwell R. Adjuvant drugs for postoperative pain management. Current Anaesthesia and Critical Care 1995;6:81-86

ANSWER 69

A. TRUE   B. FALSE   C. TRUE   D. FALSE   E. FALSE

Red blood cell survival is defined as greater than 70% survival at 24 hours after transfusion. This is 35 days for SAG-M stored blood which has an Hct of 0.6-0.7. At 7 days coagulation factors V and VIII have almost disappeared and IX, X, and XI are reduced.

Ref: Yentis SM. Anaesthesia A to Z. Blood storage.

ANSWER 70

A. TRUE   B. FALSE   C. TRUE   D. FALSE   E. FALSE

Cerebral ischaemia occurs when intracranial pressure acutely rises via compression of cerebral blood vessels. There is an abrupt increase in sympathetic nervous system traffic and blood pressure rises. The heart rate falls by a secondary reflex via the baroreceptors. The coronary chemoreceptor reflex, the Bezold Jarish reflex, can result clinically from coronary angiography and myocardial necrosis - possibly during an inferior myocardial infarction. The arterial baroreceptors are more active in their response to falls in blood pressure than to rises. Distension of atriae or vena cavae produces vagal impulses which lead to a reflex tachycardia, the Bainbridge reflex. This will be abolished by vagotomy. The arterial baroreceptors reset to a raised blood pressure within hours and then continue to function on an acute basis. They have little role in the long term control of blood pressure.

Ref: Priebe and Skarvan. Cardiovascular Physiology. Chapter 6. Cardiovascular control mechanisms.

ANSWER 71

A. FALSE   B. TRUE   C. FALSE   D. FALSE   E. TRUE

Renal potassium excretion is governed by aldosterone and by acid-base status. Hydrogen ions can compete with potassium ions for exchange with sodium in the renal tubule. Systemic acidosis results in hyperkalaemia and alkalosis in hypokalaemia. Common stimuli and diseases that alter aldosterone secretion are:-

INCREASE: Hyperkalaemia, Angiotensin II (increased by:-heart failure, cirrhosis, poor renal function eg RAS, Conn's Sx)

DECREASE: Hypokalaemia, Heparin, NSAID, Hyporeninaemic hypoaldosteronism, Hypoadrenalism

Ref Current Anaesthesia and Critical Care 1996; Vol 7, No 4: pg 176-181. Physiology and pathophysiology of fluids and electrolytes.

ANSWER 72

A. TRUE   B. FALSE   C. TRUE   D. FALSE   E. FALSE

The Cochrane group in Oxford is one of the groups looking into evidence based medicine. It is not a financially driven exercise but an attempt to identify best therapy. Literature is divided into four classes and best therapy is then illucidated. A simple question in anaesthetic practice could be "Which antiemetic agents should be prescribed post surgery?"

ANSWER 73

A. TRUE   B. TRUE   C. FALSE   D. TRUE   E TRUE

Hypokalaemia is caused by reduced intake; tissue redistribution (including insulin, salbutamol, B12 therapy); increased gastrointestinal loss (including diarrhoea, vomiting, NG suction); and increased renal loss (including diuretics, hyperaldosteronism, renal artery stenosis, hypomagnesaemia, polyuric renal failure). Hypokalaemia causes anorexia, nausea, muscle weakness, paralytic ileus and most importantly cardiac conduction abnormalities. Rhabdomyolysis causes hyperkalaemia.

Ref: Turner, D.A.B. (1990) Fluid, electrolyte and acid-base balance. In: Aitkenhead, A.R. and Smith, G. (Eds.) Textbook of Anaesthesia, 2nd edn. pp. 389-404. Edinburgh: Churchill Livingstone

ANSWER 74

A. TRUE   B. FALSE   C. FALSE   D. TRUE   E FALSE

The only absolute indications for one lung anaesthesia are

1. Isolation from infection or massive haemorrhage

2. Control of ventilation during surgery for bronchopleural fistulae, unilateral cyst and tracheobronchial rupture. All other indications are relative.

Ref: Miller RD. Anesthesia 3rd ed. Churchill Livingstone. Ch 50.

ANSWER 75

A. FALSE   B. FALSE   C. FALSE   D. FALSE   E. TRUE

The standard surgical tracheostomy was described in 1909. Since 1985, the Ciaglia technique has increased in popularity and other techniques including using dilator forceps and the trans-laryngeal approach are also used. Timing of tracheostomy can follow guidelines, but should be individualised to the patient. The patient is positioned with the neck extended and one experienced physician provides sedation and care of the existing artificial airway. The skin and trachea are punctured, after the endotracheal tube has been withdrawn (usually so that the cuff lies just inferior to the vocal cords), at the level of the first or second tracheal interspace. A guidewire is inserted and the tract is dilated using graduated dilators until the tracheostomy tube can be inserted. Some operators use a skin incision and/or blunt dissection to aid dilatation. Immediate complications include bleeding, paratracheal insertion, pneumothorax, subcutaneous emphysema, hypoxia, hypotension, loss of airway and death. Both puncture of the endotracheal tube cuff and obstruction of its lumen with a bronchoscope (used to aid safety) can result in a reduction in minute volume. Complications occurring due to the tracheostomy tube include bleeding, infection, tube displacement or obstruction, cuff leakage, tracheal erosion, transoesophageal fistula and death. Long term complications include cosmetic deformity, tracheal granuloma, tracheomalacia and laryngeal stenosis. The incidence of these compares favourably with surgical tracheostomies.

Ref: Friedman Y. Indications, timing, techniques, and complications of tracheostomy in the critically ill patient. Current Opinion in Critical Care 1996;2:47-53

ANSWER 76

A. FALSE   B. TRUE   C. FALSE   D. TRUE   E. FALSE

Entonox is supplied in size D, F, and G cylinders. Its international standard cylinder colours are blue and white as for its United Kingdom storage. Its pseudocritical temperature is -6°C and therefore it can be stored down to 0°C. However if separation does occur both warming and inversion/rotation of cylinders in suggested. The entonox valve does fit directly onto the pin index system however it is a two stage system of regulator and demand valve.

Ref: Ward. Anaesthetic equipment. Chapter 8. Intermittent flow and on-demand apparatus.
Ref: Craft and Upton. Key topics in Anaesthesia. Nitrous oxide. Supply of anaesthetic gases.

ANSWER 77

A. FALSE   B. FALSE   C. FALSE   D. FALSE   E. TRUE

The transport environment is hostile and diagnosis of new conditions is difficult, and so transport should not occur until the patient has been stabilised (including surgery) and fully assessed. Apart from ECG and SaO_2, IBP is highly desirable due to the intermittent recordings and failure rate of non-invasive methods. Palpated heart rate has been shown to be closely correlated to that measured from an ECG, but dysrhythmias and changes in ECG morphology are missed. Hypovolaemic paients tolerate transfer poorly and cardiac filling pressure measurements are advisabe in those with difficult to assess volume status. Intubation with ventilation is needed in any case of prospective respiratory failure or obstruction/aspiration. Well prepared patients can be transported safely by road and will avoid the specific dangers of aeromedical transfer (air space enlargement, reduced oxygen partial pressure, accelerative forces which affect heart rate less if the paient lies across the axis of the force on motion). Monitors must be compact and have adequate battery life. Don't forget drugs and an adequate supply of oxygen. It is safest to assume a worst case scenario e.g. 100% oxygen requirements at supranormal minute ventilation in a transfer delayed to at least double its predicted length of time. Size E oxygen cylinders hold 680 litres when full.

Ref: Runcie CJ, Reeve W, Reidy J, Wallace PGM. Secondary transport of the critically ill adult. Clinical Intensive Care 1991;2:217-225

ANSWER 78

A. TRUE   B. TRUE   C. TRUE   D. TRUE   E. TRUE

In pericarditis the chest pain is often pleuritic and ST elevation occurs in all leads except aVR. Oesophageal rupture should be considered when chest pain follows violent vomiting and/or is associated with surgical emphysema above the clavicle. A tension pneumothorax may present with chest pain, shock, right bundle branch block and dyspnoea. A widened mediastinum on erect chest X-ray is indicative of thoracic aortic dissection. Both pulmonary emboli and myocardial infarction may lead to right bundle branch block or T wave inversion in anterolateral ECG leads and a similar clinical picture.

Ref: Weatherall, Ledingham & Warrell. Oxford Textbook of Medicine. vol2 section 13

ANSWER 79

A. FALSE   B. FALSE   C. TRUE   D. FALSE   E. TRUE

The femoral nerve (L2 to L4) arises from the lumbar plexus. It descends in the pelvis in the groove between psoas and iliacus and enters the thigh deep to the inguinal ligament. Here it lies lateral to the femoral artery and vein. It supplies skin to the anterior and medial aspect of the thigh. Its branches include anterior and medial femoral cutaneous and saphenous nerves.

It is the common peroneal nerve (a branch of the sciatic) that winds around the neck of the fibula and hence maybe damaged in fractures here.

Ref. Lumley, Craven and Aitken. Essential Anatomy and Some Clinical Applications. Churchill Livingstone.

ANSWER 80

A. FALSE   B. TRUE   C. FALSE   D. FALSE   E. TRUE

Loss of enteral nutrition changes the gut structure and function, this includes villous atrophy, reduced gut mucosal barrier integrity and impaired release of gut trophic hormones. Beneficial effects of enteral feeding include reduced frequency of stress ulceration and gall bladder emptying. In a meta-analysis comparing 8 trials of enteral vs parenteral feeding the frequency of septic complications was halved in patients fed enterally. As well as less pancreatic exocrine secretion, elemental feeds do not promote intestinal growth factors to the same extent as more complex feeds and so cause or perpetuate gut atrophy. The duration of surgery and amount of bowel handling at laparotomy do not correlate with the duration of ileus. Hyponatremia, hypokalaemia, hypocalcaemia and hypomagnesaemia can all cause paralytic ileus and hypomagnesaemia is often overlooked. The frequency of diarrhoea in the ICU patient being enterally fed is approximately 60% compared with 25% in the non-ICU patient and is multifactorial. The commonest causes include antibiotics, lack of enteral feeding, hypoalbuminaemia, infected feed, intolerance of the osmotic load, lactose intolerance and inappropriate laxative therapy. Most ICUs deliver enteral nuitrition by continuous feeding rather than bolus administration. This reduces gastrointestinal side-effects but may lead to increased gram negative colonisation of the upper GI tract as the continuous presence of feed in the stomach may buffer gastric acidity and its bactericidal effect. The strategy of discontinuing the feed for a time to allow a decrease in gastric pH has been shown to reduce the incidence of gram negative pulmonary infection. Most units feed for 18-20 hours continuously and then have a 4-6 hour break, usually at night.

Ref: Current Anaesthesia and Critical Care. 1996; Vol 7, No 2: pg 62-76. The role of the gut in critical illness & enteral nutrition.

ANSWER 81

A. TRUE   B. TRUE   C. FALSE   D. TRUE   E. TRUE

Binding of basic drugs is unaffected in renal failure, however acidic drugs which mainly bind to albumin may be significantly affected by hypoalbuminaemia. Uraemia leads to conformational changes in receptors and competition for binding sites caused by drug accumulation. The critical creatinine clearance in terms of extending drug half lives is 10-20 ml/min. Phenothiazine clearance is unchanged in renal failure.

Ref: Belani KG. Kidney transplantation. International Anesthesiology Clinics 29. Lippcott. pp17-39 1991

ANSWER 82

A. TRUE   B. FALSE   C. TRUE   D. FALSE   E. TRUE

The trunks of the brachial plexus branch beneath the clavicle. The anterior branches of the upper and middle trunks then unite to form a common or outer cord. The anterior branch of the lower trunk forms the inner cord. The posterior branches of all three trunks form the posterior cord. These cords run alongside the axillary artery. In the neck the brachial plexus lies in the posterior triangle and is covered by skin, platysma and deep fascia. The median nerve arises from the inner and outer cords of the brachial plexus. The circumflex nerve courses around the surgical neck of humerus and is liable to be damaged in fractures or dislocations of the humerus. This will lead to paralysis of deltoid.

Ref. Pick and Howden. Gray's Anatomy. Galley Press.

ANSWER 83

A. FALSE   B. FALSE   C. FALSE   D. FALSE   E. TRUE

The UK code of practice requires the diagnosis of brain stem death be made by two medical practitioners who have experience in the field. At least one must be a consultant; the other may be an SR (the situation regarding SpRs has not been clarified). Earlier statements by the Conference of Medical Royal Colleges had required that they be registered for 5 years but this does not form part of the 1981 recommendations. The only requirement in terms of the timing of the second set of tests is that 'the interval should be adequate for the reassurance of all those directly concerned'. It appears that 2-3 hours is considered sufficient. In the UK the time of death is at the conclusion of the second set of tests, not when the heart stops beating or is removed as in Denmark. The EEG does not form part of the UK criteria since an isoelectric EEG does not exclude neurological recovery following cerebral ischaemia and some cortical activity can be detected in patients with complete brain stem disruption.

Ref: Current Anaesthesia and Critical Care 1994; Vol 5, No 1: pg36-40. The diagnosis and management of brain death.

ANSWER 84

A. FALSE   B. TRUE   C. TRUE   D. FALSE   E. TRUE

The mucous membrane of the larynx is supplied by the internal laryngeal nerve above the vocal cords and the recurrent laryngeal nerve below. The cricothyroid muscle is supplied by the external laryngeal nerve. The other musles of the larynx (posterior and lateral cricoarytenoid, transverse arytenoid, ary-epiglottic and thyroarytenoid) are supplied by the recurrent laryngeal nerve. The vocal cords are lined by stratified squamous epithelium, the larynx above and the lower part of the larynx are lined by respiratory epithelium. The larynx is raised by the palatopharyngeus, sapingopharyngeus, stylopharyngeus and thyrohyoid. It is lowered by the infrahyoid muscle aided by gravity. Within the larynx 2 pairs of parallel horizontal folds are present in the lateral walls. The upper is the vestibular fold (false vocal cord), the lower is the true vocal cord. The gap between the vocal folds is known as the rima glottidis.

Ref. Lumley, Craven and Aitken. Essential Anatomy and Some Clinical Applications. Churchill Livingstone.

ANSWER 85

A. TRUE   **B. FALSE**   **C. TRUE**   **D. FALSE**   **E. FALSE**

Air embolus may occur when the venous pressure is lower than atmospheric pressure. It occurs when an open vein is above heart level. It is particularly likely in the sitting position during neurosurgery since the dural sinuses do not collapse. Air emboli trapped in the lung will increase dead space and so cause a fall in end-tidal carbon dioxide. Obstruction to right sided heart filling will raise the central venous pressure. The left lateral head down position is recommended on diagnosis. This prevents a large embolus from entering the pulmonary artery by trapping it in the right ventricle. Trans-oesophageal echo is the most sensitive means of detecting emboli, it is however non-specific, being unable to differentiate between air, fat and blood microemboli.

Ref: Craft & Upton. Key Topics in Anaesthesia. Bios Scientific Publishers.

ANSWER 86

A. FALSE   **B. FALSE**   **C. TRUE**   **D. TRUE**   **E. TRUE**

The EEG is scalp recorded summated post synaptic action potentials. They are relatively closely related to cerebral blood flow and oxygen consumption. The voltages are small (10-100 microvolts), and low impedance electrodes (usually chlorided silver discs) are required. Certain frequency bands have been traditionally described to help in diagnosis. Alpha activity is 8-13 Hz, beta is above 13 Hz, theta is 4-7 Hz and delta is below 4 Hz. Barbiturates initially increase fast activity but as the dose increases, the slower frequency bands become more prominent. As the level increases further, burst suppression occurs (high voltage, low frequency activity alternating with electrical silence) and finally there is loss of all electrical activity. The ECG can be monitored by the EEG and this is used to compare activity with the heart rate.

Ref: Sykes, Vickers and Hull. Principles of Measurement and Monitoring in Anaesthesia and Intensive Care. Blackwell Scientific Publications. Ch 24.

ANSWER 87

A. FALSE   **B. FALSE**   **C. FALSE**   **D. TRUE**   **E. FALSE**

Paracetamol is metabolised by two hepatic pathways. Glucuronide or sulphate conjugation is harmless. Metabolism by the mixed function oxidase system produces a toxic metabolite that is rendered harmless by glutathione. 10 grammes (20 tablets) of paracetamol is enough to deplete liver glutathione and leave the toxic metabolite to damage sulphydryl groups of hepatic enzymes and cause centrilobular necrosis. The toxic metabolite is produced in larger quantities following induction of the mixed function oxidase enzyme system, thus increasing the likelihood of paracetamol toxicity occuring. Right upper quadrant abdominal pain, nausea and vomiting are features within 24 hours of ingestion. In the next 24 hours most patients recover fully. Loss of consciousness is not a feature at this time. N-acetyl cysteine offers the best protection when given less than 10 hours after ingestion and it offers some protection up to 15 hours after, but after this time it gives no protection. Elevation of the prothrombin time is the best guide to severity.

Ref: Kumar & Clark. Clinical Medicine. Balliere Tindall.

ANSWER   88

A. FALSE   B. FALSE   C. FALSE   D. TRUE   E. FALSE

The following are the correct anatomical levels.

The cricoid cartilage : the sixth cervical vertebra.

The body of the hyoid bone : the body of the third cervical vertebra.

The upper border of the thyroid cartilage : the body of the fourth cervical vertebra.

The isthmus of the thyroid gland : between the second to the fourth tracheal rings.

The thoracic termination of the trachea : the body of the fourth thoracic vertebra (sternal angle).

Ref. Snell. Clinical Anatomy For Medical Students. Little Brown. Boston.

ANSWER   89

A. FALSE   B. FALSE   C. TRUE   D. FALSE   E. FALSE

ARF from whatever cause is characterised by a rapid loss of renal function with the retention of urea, creatinine, hydrogen ions and other metabolic products. Oliguria (< 400 ml urine / 24 hrs) is only present in about 50% of patients with ARF and isolated values of serum electrolytes do not differentiate between the various patho-physiological causes. Classically ARF is described as being pre-renal, intrinsic or post-renal in origin. Biochemical values that aim to distinguish between pre-renal and intrinsic ARF are:-

	pre-renal	intrinsic
Urine sodium concentration	< 20 mmol/l	> 40 mmol/l
Urine:serum urea concentration	> 10:1	< 3:1
Urine:serum osmolality	> 1.5:1	< 1.1:1

Ref: Marshall. Gower Medical Publishing. Clinical Chemistry. Ch 5 Renal Disorders.

ANSWER   90

A. FALSE   B. TRUE   C. TRUE   D. TRUE   E. FALSE

Although a left atrial pressure of 18 mmHg is greater than normal it has been found to be the optimum for left ventricular performance in patients with shock from recent MIs and anything less is consistent with hypovolaemia. The aim of catecholamine therapy is to increase arterial pressure and improve coronary perfusion. This increased pressure is, however, at the expense of increased myocardial oxygen consumption which may endanger additional areas of myocardium. Comparisons between dopamine and dobutamine in patients with low output states have shown dobutamine to be superior. The potential benefits of vasodilator therapy include a reduction in myocardial work and oxygen demand; reduction in atrial pressures due to venous pooling of blood; redistribution of organ blood flow. However, vasodilators tend to increase hypoxaemia by increasing intrapulmonary shunting. Salbutamol is a relatively specific beta-2 agonist and its main effect is arteriolar dilatation and in patients with cardiogenic shock it can increase cardiac output without affecting PCWP.

Ref: T.E. OH. Intensive Care Manual. Butterworths. 3rd Ed. Ch 59 Cardiogenic shock

Exam 4

QUESTION 1

Concerning the maintenance of body temperature

A. The reflex responses activated by cold are controlled from the anterior hypothalamus
B. Interleukin-1 release results in fever production
C. 10% of body heat is lost from the respiratory tract
D. Thyroid stimulating hormone (TSH) secretion is increased by heat
E. The anti-pyretic effect of aspirin is exerted directly on the hypothalamus

QUESTION 2

The following are normal nutritional parameters for a 70 kg man who is not hypercatabolic

A. Carbohydrate reserve of 0.5 kg, mainly as liver glycogen
B. 24 hour caloric requirement of 2450 – 2800 kcal (10,150 – 11,900 kJ)
C. 24 hour nitrogen requirement of 10 gm
D. Protein reserve of 4 – 6 kg, mainly in muscle
E. A calorie:nitrogen ratio of 80:1

QUESTION 3

In a patient with severe aortic stenosis undergoing a general anaesthetic

A. There is a direct relationship between calculated aortic valve area and blood flow across the valve
B. A peak aortic valve gradient of 30 mmHg is not compatible with the diagnosis
C. A faster heart rate will be important to help left ventricular filling
D. A reduction in systemic vascular resistance has little effect on ventricular emptying
E. Episodes of myocardial ischaemia should be treated with GTN

QUESTION 4

Oesophageal Doppler Monitoring

A. Is of value for measuring blood flow
B. Can be used to measure left atrial pressure
C. Allows monitoring of the left ventricular wall motion
D. Relies on measuring the aortic diameter to calculate cardiac output
E. As a measure of cardiac output has been successfully validated by comparison with thermodilution

QUESTION 5

In the patient with an ejection systolic murmur

A. The patient with aortic stenosis has an increased risk of perioperative mortality
B. Two dimensional echocardiography is used to assess gradient across the valve
C. Aortic gradients greater than 25 mmHg are regarded as significant
D. The patient will require antibiotic cover perioperatively
E. An aortic gradient less than 50 mmHg excludes severe aortic stenosis

QUESTION 6

Subdural haematomas

A. Arise from middle meningeal artery haemorrhage
B. Are always unilateral
C. Are more common than extradural haematomas
D. Can be associated with minor trauma
E. Have a good prognosis from surgery if mid brain coning has not occurred

QUESTION 7

Neonates

A. Lose up to 10% of their birth weight in the first few days of life
B. Have double the cardiac output per kg of adults
C. Are unable to perceive pain at a cortical level
D. Are more susceptible to opioid induced apnoea if premature
E. Should be given NSAIDs in preference to opioids whenever possible

QUESTION 8

Concerning hypovolaemic shock

A. It only occurs when the reduction in circulating blood volume is greater than 40%
B. There is a depletion of cellular adenosine triphosphate (ATP)
C. As it progresses capillary permeability increases
D. Hyperventilation occurs due to central chemoreceptor stimulation
E. Hepatic arterial but not portal venous blood flow is reduced

QUESTION 9

Torsades de pointes may be caused by

A. Quinidine
B. Amitryptyline
C. Aspirin
D. Hyperkalaemia
E. Erythromycin

QUESTION 10

A successful stellate ganglion block may cause

A. Ipsilateral miosis
B. Contralateral nasal congestion
C. Bilateral ptosis
D. Ipsilateral exomphalos
E. Horners syndrome

QUESTION 11

Clinical features of iron deficiency anaemia include

A. Koilonychia
B. Glossitis
C. Brittle hair
D. Dysphagia
E. Parotid gland enlargement

QUESTION 12

In the event of a traumatic injury to a limb

A. Compartment syndrome will not occur if a fracture is open
B. The presence of a bruit suggests arterial injury
C. Calcaneal fractures are associated with vertebral injury
D. An amputated digit remains viable for reimplantation for 24 hours
E. Involving the median nerve, sensation to the little finger is lost

QUESTION 13

Neurolept malignant syndrome

A. Is a mild form of malignant hyperpyrexia (MH)
B. Causes rhabdomyolysis
C. Can be triggered by the use of bromocriptine
D. Is associated with a low grade temperature (<38°C)
E. Does not respond to the administration of dantrolene

QUESTION 14

Considering the functioning of enzymes

A. The rate of an enzymatically controlled process can be described by the Michaelis Menten equation

B. If a high concentration of substrate is present the rate of reaction will be proportional to the enzyme concentration

C. Catecholamines do not utilise a second messenger

D. Cyclic AMP is the intracellular second messenger for ACTH

E. Calcium ions entering into cells can bind to calmodulin which then acts as a second messenger

QUESTION 15

Duodenal perforation

A. Is less common than gastric perforation

B. May present with symptoms resembling acute appendicitis

C. Causes an increased serum amylase

D. Absence of free gas beneath the diaphragm on erect chest X-ray excludes the diagnosis

E. Contra-indicates the use of a gastrograffin swallow

QUESTION 16

The following congenital conditions cause cyanosis

A. Fallots tetralogy

B. Transposition of the great arteries

C. Coarctation

D. Patent ductus arteriosus

E. Totally anomalous pulmonary venous drainage

QUESTION 17

In the case of closed abdominal injury

A. The liver is the organ most frequently injured

B. The presence of > 1000 red cells / mm^3 of peritoneal lavage fluid is an indication for laparotomy

C. Computerised tomography is less sensitive than peritoneal lavage at detecting intra-peritoneal blood

D. Partial splenic resection is an alternative to splenectomy

E. Road traffic accidents account for most significant injuries

QUESTION 18

Haemodynamic changes associated with abdominal aortic cross-clamping include

A. Reduction in stroke volume
B. Redistribution of blood from the inferior vena cava to the superior vena cava
C. Decreased venous return
D. Increased systemic vascular resistance
E. Decreased arterial blood pressure

QUESTION 19

When comparing corticosteroid activity

A. Dexamethasone 4 mg = Hydrocortisone 20 mg
B. Prednisolone 5 mg = Methylprednisolone 4 mg
C. Dexamethasone has less mineralocorticoid activity than hydrocortisone
D. Prednisolone is more potent than betamethasone
E. Sodium retention is less likely with methylprednisolone than hydrocortisone

QUESTION 20

Post gastrectomy complications include

A. Bilious vomiting
B. Hypoglycaemia
C. Diarrhoea
D. Intestinal obstruction
E. Attacks of flushing

QUESTION 21

Side effects of methyl dopa treatment include

A. Sedation
B. Bradycardia
C. Diarrhoea
D. Haemolytic anaemia
E. Gynaecomastia

QUESTION 22

The following are therapeutic plasma concentrations

A. Aminophylline 18 mg/litre
B. Diazepam 50 mcg/litre
C. Digoxin 4 mcg/litre
D. Phenytoin 15 mg/litre
E. Lignocaine 6 mg/litre

QUESTION 23

In the coronary circulation

A. Increased oxygen demand is mainly met by increased oxygen extraction
B. Lactate is a significant energy supply during exercise
C. During coronary artery disease collaterals develop in the endocardium
D. Endothelin and nitric oxide exist in vasoconstrictor and vasodilator balance
E. Significant right coronary artery perfusion occurs during systole

QUESTION 24

When monitoring TO4 with a peripheral nerve stimulator

A. Delivered current should be 50% greater than the threshold for maximal stimulation
B. Most nerve stimulators deliver a fixed pulse of 0.2 ms duration
C. Fade is minimized at a stimulus frequency of 2Hz
D. Fade is due to pre-junctional ACh receptor blockade
E. Tetanic stimulation alters the response for up to 30 mins

QUESTION 25

In patients with chronic obstructive pulmonary disease (COPD)

A. Hyperphosphataemia results in increased respiratory muscle weakness
B. Tidal volume is increased
C. Gas trapping during positive pressure ventilation increases the risk of ventilator induced lung injury
D. A high fat diet can increase the work required to maintain $PaCO_2$
E. Normal arterial blood gases should be aimed for if positive pressure ventilation is commenced

QUESTION 26

In acute pancreatitis

A. Serum amylase levels correlate with severity
B. Mumps is a causative factor
C. Hypercalcaemia can result
D. Adult respiratory distress is a complication
E. Total parenteral nutrition helps reduce the amount of enzyme in the gland

QUESTION 27

In a patient with peptic ulceration

- **A.** Acid secretion is greater in those with gastric ulceration than those with duodenal ulceration
- **B.** Diarrhoea is a side effect of treatment with aluminium salts
- **C.** Hyperparathyroidism is a cause
- **D.** Duodenal ulcer pain classically occurs at night
- **E.** Ranitidine is more successful in the treatment of duodenal ulcer than gastric ulcer

QUESTION 28

In a 4 week old neonate with pyloric stenosis

- **A.** The urine can be concentrated up to 600 mOsm/l
- **B.** A paradoxically alkaline urine will occur
- **C.** Hyponatraemia only occurs later in the metabolic disturbances
- **D.** Any hypochloraemia is worsened by further renal chloride loss
- **E.** Any hypokalaemia is partly due to intracellular redistribution

QUESTION 29

Causes of an increased end expiratory PCO_2 during anaesthesia include

- **A.** Hyperthermia
- **B.** Complete airway obstruction
- **C.** Hypotension
- **D.** Air embolism
- **E.** Sodium bicarbonate infusion

QUESTION 30

Metabolic acidosis with an elevated anion gap is associated with

- **A.** Distal renal tubular acidosis
- **B.** Glucose-6-phosphatase deficiency
- **C.** Ileostomy
- **D.** Botulism
- **E.** Diabetic ketoacidosis

QUESTION 31

Concerning informed consent for surgery

A. In England the patient should be over the age of 16

B. Verbal consent is inadequate

C. In mental illness, consent is usually sought from the Courts

D. Life saving surgery may proceed when consent is unobtainable

E. Is valid if given once the patient has been premedicated

QUESTION 32

Sevoflurane

A. Is an isomer of isoflurane

B. Induces cardiovascular stimulation when the inspired concentration is rapidly increased

C. Increases intracranial pressure

D. Is converted to compound A more readily at higher temperatures

E. Anaesthesia does not cause a rise in serum fluoride concentration

QUESTION 33

Magnetic resonance imaging (MRI)

A. Relies on the radiofrequency radiation emitted by an unpaired electron exposed to pulses of radiofrequency radiation

B. Carbon-12 is an atom that is detected by MRI

C. Infusion devices can be safely placed at the edge of the fringe field

D. Is the technique of choice to image the posterior fossa

E. Requires the use of Hydrogen-2 in a contrast medium to enhance the scans

QUESTION 34

Status epilepticus

A. Is defined as seizures occurring within 5 minutes of each other

B. Has a mortality of 40%

C. Is a contraindication to the use of atracurium

D. Lasting beyond 1 hour in a child is associated with a 65% chance of permanent neurological morbidity

E. Should be treated with thiopentone if diazepam does not control fitting

QUESTION 35

Multiple uptake gated acquisition

A. Uses thallium-201 labelled red blood cells
B. Divides the cardiac cycle into 30-50 ms intervals
C. Is a reliable indicator of myocardial contractility
D. Preoperative data has been shown to correlate with early perioperative infarction
E. Is used in combination with dipyridamole to demonstrate "steal"

QUESTION 36

Pulse Oximetry

A. Reduces post-operative complications
B. Decreases the incidence of myocardial ischaemia
C. Is accurate to 0.2% at a saturation of 95%
D. A sudden fall in SaO_2 will show no change in SpO_2 for 15 seconds at least
E. Relies on the Hoppe-Seyler Law of light transmission

QUESTION 37

Portal hypertension

A. Occurs secondary to tricuspid incompetence
B. Is a contraindication to extradural blockade
C. Is associated with Budd-Chiari syndrome
D. Leads to hypoalbuminaemia
E. Causes thrombocytosis

QUESTION 38

The stress response to surgery

A. Can be modified using opioids
B. Is the result of sympathetic nervous system stimulation
C. Is modified to a very small degree by intravenous anaesthetic agents
D. Is more pronounced when patients breathe spontaneously
E. Is reduced by the addition of PEEP

QUESTION 39

The measurement of gastric mucosal pH (pHi)

A. Is inaccurate if the patient is fasting
B. Should be preceded by the administration of a drug to prevent gastric acid secretion
C. Is predictive of morbidity and mortality in the perioperative period
D. Involves introducing air into a silicone balloon on the end of a nasogastric tube
E. Requires the measurement of arterial bicarbonate concentration

QUESTION 40

Tramadol

A. Has preferential activity at mu opioid receptors

B. Analgesia can be reversed fully by naloxone

C. Is presented as a racemic mixture of two enantiomers

D. Is useful for the treatment of postoperative pain as the incidence of nausea is less than 10%

E. Inhibits 5-hydoxytryptamine (5-HT) reuptake

QUESTION 41

Nitric oxide

A. Is an endothelial derived relaxing factor (EDRF)

B. Is synthesised from the amino acid L-citrulline

C. Is the active moiety of glyceryl trinitrate

D. Can cause prolongation of the prothrombin time when administered by the inhaled method in acute lung injury

E. Production can be reduced by the administration of citrulline

QUESTION 42

Chronic pancreatitis

A. Can present with recurrent steatorrhoea

B. Causes death in 70% within 5 years

C. Is unrelated to alcohol intake

D. Occurs post trauma

E. Occurs as a complication of cystic fibrosis

QUESTION 43

Regarding hyperbaric oxygen therapy

A. It is the only method by which arterial PaO_2 can exceed 50 kPa

B. Oxygen induced vasoconstriction may limit tissue oxygen levels in some organs

C. It allows tissue oxygen requirements to be met from dissolved oxygen

D. It is still used to prolong the period of circulatory arrest safely

E. It is useful in the treatment of severe anaerobic infections

QUESTION 44

Concerning capnography

A. Mainstream and sidestream capnographs use infra-red light absorption to measure CO_2
B. Sidestream analysis uses low aspiration rates from the circuit to increase carbon dioxide sensitivity
C. It reliably detects endobronchial intubation
D. Both sidestream and mainstream types require water traps
E. It can cause burns

QUESTION 45

The following poisons are paired with their specific antidotes

A. Propranolol   -   glucagon
B. Ethylene glycol - methanol
C. Lead   -   penicillamine
D. Paraquat   -   pralidoxime
E. Theophylline   -   propranolol

QUESTION 46

Risk factors for developing acute renal failure (ARF) include

A. Normal pregnancy
B. Nephrotic syndrome
C. Myeloma
D. Chronic liver disease
E. Peripheral vascular disease

QUESTION 47

Clubbing is seen in

A. Ulcerative colitis
B. Cirrhosis
C. Myxoedema
D. Fallots tetralogy
E. Acromegaly

QUESTION 48

The following principles apply when patients with major trauma require anaesthesia

A. The central volume of distribution is decreased resulting in greater drug effects
B. Rocuronium bromide causes less rise in intracranial or intraocular pressure than suxamethonium
C. Narcotic analgesics aggravate shock and increase sympathetic tone
D. The uptake of volatile anaesthetic agents is increased
E. The incidence of awarenes during anaesthesia has been shown to be in excess of 30%

QUESTION 49

In the management of a patient having elective hypotensive anaesthesia

A. Blood loss is reduced more than by lowering of cardiac output alone
B. Nitroprusside is excreted as thiocyanate in the urine
C. Nitroprusside used to reduce MAP to 55 mmHg also causes an increase in ICP
D. The presence of mild coronary stenoses will produce myocardial ischaemia
E. Pulmonary dead space is usually decreased if blood volume is maintained

QUESTION 50

An 8 year old child weighing 25 Kg has lost 350 ml of blood in an RTA, the following are the expected physiological effects

A. Normal blood pressure
B. Anuria
C. Peripheral cyanosis
D. Tachycardia
E. Dulled response to pain

QUESTION 51

Ephedrine is unlikely to be effective in reversing hypotension in patients chronically receiving the following medication

A. Reserpine
B. Alpha–methyl dopa
C. Phenoxybenzamine
D. Clonidine
E. Propranolol

QUESTION 52

Considering the function of anaesthetic machine flowmeters

A. Individual flow meter tubes do not have to be calibrated for temperature
B. Back pressure on a flowmeter tube can cause inaccuracy
C. Position of oxygen in relation to other gases is internationally regulated
D. Static electricity may disturb flowmeter function
E. The pressure drop across the rotameter float depends on gas density and float length in a tapered tube

QUESTION 53

Causes of a raised serum alkaline phosphatase include

A. Pagets disease of bone
B. Malignant disease
C. Pregnancy
D. Myocardial infarction
E. Osteoporosis

QUESTION 54

Fibrosis of the lung is seen in

A. Fibrosing alveolitis
B. Scleroderma
C. Previous radiotherapy
D. Berylliosis
E. Organophosphorus compound poisoning

QUESTION 55

For the re-use of patient contact anaesthetic equipment

A. Autoclaving involves the use of steam at above 100°C
B. Disinfection kills all bacteria, spores, and viruses
C. Prion particles are removed by sterilisation
D. Previously irradiated pvc objects can be re-sterilised safely using ethylene oxide
E. Pseudomonas can grow in chlorhexidine solution

QUESTION 56

Contraindications to local anaesthesia for eye surgery include

A. Glaucoma
B. Inability to lie flat
C. Procedures that last more than 90 minutes
D. Penetrating eye injury
E. Retinal detachment

QUESTION 57

During the early stages of septic shock

A. There is relative hypovolaemia
B. There is absolute hypovolaemia
C. Profound vasodilatation means that vasopressors are a first line treatment
D. Dextrose saline is appropriate for use in the resuscitative phase
E. Cardiac output falls dramatically

QUESTION 58

In rheumatoid arthritis

A. Coronary arteritis is a feature
B. Symmetrical polyarthritis is a feature
C. Pulmonary fibrosis leads to an obstructive respiratory pattern
D. Renal impairment is due solely to amyloidosis
E. The skin is hypertrophic and so difficult to cannulate

QUESTION 59

Considering the risks of gastric regurgitation and aspiration

A. The lower oesophageal spincter remains competent at intragastric pressures of <20 cmH$_2$0
B. Sodium citrate 0.3M 30 ml orally raises the gastric pH for 1-3 hours
C. Ranitidine 150mg orally achieves therapeutic plasma levels for 8 hours
D. Suxamethonium causes a decrease in barrier pressure
E. Pulmonary damage increases proportionately as the pH of any aspirate decreases below 2.5

QUESTION 60

Concerning the management of patients with the acquired immune deficiency syndrome (AIDS)

A. There is impaired cell mediated immunity due to a deficiency of CD8+ B-cells
B. Some patients have defects of antibody-mediated immune responses
C. Recurrent respiratory tract infections with Haemophilus influenzae, Pneumococcus or Pseudomonas are common
D. The main side-effect of zidovudine is myelosuppression
E. Ventilatory support is contraindicated in Pneumocystis carinii pneumonia

QUESTION 61

Visceral Pain

A. Referred pain is felt in the cutaneous area corresponding to the dorsal horn neurone upon which the visceral afferents converge
B. Is poorly localised
C. Referred pain may be associated with allodynia and hyperalgesia
D. Is commonly associated with nausea
E. Afferents from the small intestine reach the spinal cord at the same level as those from the urinary bladder

QUESTION 62

Regarding the use of patient-controlled analgesia (PCA) for post-operative pain relief

A. Patients using PCA require significantly less opioid than those receiving IM opioids
B. Intrathecal opioids provide superior analgesia
C. Respiratory depression occurs 10 times less commonly than with continuous infusions
D. The personnel time required for PCA related activities is 20% less than that required for IM analgesia activities
E. The incidence of mishaps during PCA therapy is 12%

QUESTION 63

Bacterial meningitis

A. Is most commonly caused by Streptococcus pneumonii in UK
B. Results in an elevated CSF glucose
C. Results in an elevated CSF protein content
D. Can be associated with pericarditis
E. Vaccine is available for Meningococci groups A and C

QUESTION 64

The following mediators are commonly released or activated during septicemic shock and multiple organ failure

A. Complement fragments
B. Bradykinin
C. Serotonin
D. Thrombomodulin
E. Alpha 2 macroglobulin

QUESTION 65

Hypothermia causes the following physiological changes

A. Apnoea below a core temperature of 30°C
B. J waves in the ECG indicating an increased risk of ventricular fibrillation
C. Shivering which can increase basal heat production five fold
D. A 50% reduction in cardiac output at 30°C
E. Increased parasympathetic activity in the brown fat of infants

QUESTION 66

Concerning depth of anaesthesia

A. Guedels stages of anaesthesia relate to progressively deeper levels of chloroform anaesthesia
B. The conductivity of skin decreases with increasing depth of anaesthesia
C. Spontaneous lower oesophageal contractions increase with increasing depth of anaesthesia
D. A positive response with the isolated forearm is only weakly predicitive of recall
E. Cerebral function monitors provide a sensitive measure of depth of anaesthesia

QUESTION 67

Oxygenation during single lung ventilation can be improved by

A. The addition of PEEP to the collapsed lung
B. The addition of oxygen at 4 l/min to the ventilated lung
C. The addition of CPAP to the collapsed lung
D. Increasing the inspired FiO_2
E. Using inotropes to improve cardiac output

QUESTION 68

The following statements about breathing systems are true

A. In a Mapleson A system during controlled ventilation a short expiratory pause promotes rebreathing

B. In a Mapleson B system fresh gas enters the system closer to the patient than the expiratory valve

C. The Ambu E valve is suitable for use during spontaneous ventilation

D. In the T piece system the volume of the expiratory limb should be twice the patients tidal volume

E. In the Heidbrink valve, the valve should be light to avoid sticking

QUESTION 69

Concerning brachial plexus blockade

A. The interscalene approach provides for anaesthesia to the ulnar border of the forearm

B. The supraclavicular approach is not reliable to produce anaesthesia to the hand

C. The axillary approach is least likely to cause pneumothorax

D. Diaphragmatic paralysis is a complication

E. Puncture of an artery may be deliberate

QUESTION 70

When considering normal standard electrocardiography

A. The recording speed is 50 mm/s

B. The PR interval is between 3 - 5 mm squares

C. The axis lies between –30 degrees and +60 degrees

D. The T wave is less than 5 mm in height

E. Lead V6 is placed in the fifth intercostal space, anterior axillary line

QUESTION 71

In the circulation of the foetus

A. There are two umbilical veins

B. Blood flowing through the foramen ovale bypasses the left ventricle

C. The ductus arteriosus communicates between the pulmonary trunk and the aorta

D. The superior vena cava drains into the right atrium

E. The crista dividends exists in the right ventricle

QUESTION 72

During haemostasis

A. Potassium is released from platelets
B. The intrinsic pathway may be activated from rough surface contact
C. The extrinsic pathway activates factors XII, XI, IX and VIII
D. Fibrinolysis occurs
E. Thrombin activates plasminogen

QUESTION 73

Concerning the lumbar plexus

A. It is formed by anterior divisions of the four upper lumbar nerves
B. The obturator nerve is a branch
C. The iliohypogastric nerve is a branch
D. The femoral nerve lies lateral to the artery in the femoral sheath beneath the inguinal ligament
E. The ilioinguinal nerve supplies the labium majora

QUESTION 74

Central venous catheterisation

A. The tip of the cannula should be in the right atrium
B. The incidence of catheter colonisation is greater if the femoral route is used
C. The incidence of catheter-related infection is greater if the femoral route is used
D. The subclavian route is preferred for thrombocytopaenic patients
E. Giant a waves are seen in atrial fibrillation

QUESTION 75

Concerning oral anticoagulation

A. Warfarin affects the clotting factors VII, IX and XII
B. The target INR following first generation aortic valve replacement should be 2.0-3.0
C. The INR should be in the normal range for dental surgery
D. All patients with atrial fibrillation should be given anticoagulants prior to cardioversion
E. Oral warfarin is rapidly absorbed and peak plasma concentrations are achieved within 1 hour

QUESTION 76

In patients presenting for surgery with renal dysfunction

A. Thiopentone should be administered more slowly at induction
B. Ketamine is the drug of choice in patients with chronic renal failure
C. The onset of neuromuscular blockade is shortened with vecuronium
D. Cyclosporin may potentiate the action of pancuronium
E. Both morphine and pethidine have metabolites that accumulate in renal failure

QUESTION 77

The following are true about the risks of infection from blood component therapy

A. Fresh frozen plasma caries the same viral infection risk as whole blood
B. Hepatitis C is not routinely tested for in the UK
C. The risk of HIV infection is less than 1/1000000 blood transfusions in the UK
D. Fibrinogen carries a higher risk of viral infection
E. Hepatitis G is probably inactivated by plasma fractionation

QUESTION 78

When considering different modes of mechanical ventilation

A. Intermittent mandatory ventilation (IMV) always relies on patient breaths to maintain blood gas homeostasis
B. Pressure support ventilation is triggered by a spontaneous breath
C. The 'sigh' mode should be added to simulate normal physiology
D. Mandatory minute volume ensures alveolar minute volume is adequate
E. The theoretical advantage of synchronised IMV over IMV is a reduction in the work of breathing

QUESTION 79

In chronic renal failure

A. Nocturia is a feature
B. The anaemia does not respond to iron
C. The skin can be affected
D. Pericarditis can occur
E. Peripheral neuropathy is reversible with dialysis

QUESTION 80

Oesophagectomy

A. The patient may have had bowel preparation
B. The surgical approach is left thoracoabdominal
C. The surgical approach is right thoracotomy
D. The surgical approach is a right cervical incision
E. The surgical approach is upper midline laparotomy

QUESTION 81

Concerning sedation of the critically ill patient in ITU

A. 50% of patients experience anxiety or agitation
B. Haloperidol is more likely to cause hypotension than droperidol
C. The use of clonidine is limited by its tendency to cause a tachycardia
D. Benzodiazepines work by increasing chloride flux into neurones
E. Propofol has been implicated in the development of bacteraemia

QUESTION 82

Magnetic resonance imaging involves

A. The use of X-rays
B. The use of powerful magnets that are directly harmful
C. The use of magnets that are switched on and off during the scan
D. Alignment of atoms with an odd number of protons and neutrons in the patient
E. Significant heating during lengthy procedures

QUESTION 83

Concerning measurement of temperature

A. The oesophageal temperature is normally lower than rectal temperature
B. The resistance of platinum decreases with increasing temperature
C. Thermistor thermometers are used in pulmonary artery catheters
D. Smaller electrical temperature probes have a shorter response time
E. The resistance of a thermistor decrease with increasing temperature

QUESTION 84

The following tumours commonly metastasise to liver

A. Breast
B. Prostate
C. Thyroid
D. Lung
E. Testis

QUESTION 85

Cerebral Monitoring

A. The EEG may be expected to detect a 25% reduction in cerebral blood flow
B. Cerebral blood flow can be monitored by Xenon clearance
C. Transcranial doppler (TCD) may be used to monitor cerebral perfusion during carotid artery cross-clamping
D. Intracranial pressure (ICP) monitoring is useful in monitoring progress in head injured patients
E. Jugular venous monitoring helps in detection of regional hypoperfusion in the brain

QUESTION 86

The internal jugular vein

A. Begins at the jugular foramen
B. The facial vein is a tributary
C. Travels in the carotid sheath in the neck
D. Drains the scalp
E. The superior thyroid vein is a tributary

QUESTION 87

Concerning the management of the acute respiratory distress syndrome (ARDS)

A. There is evidence that efforts to achieve a negative fluid balance are associated with improved outcome
B. Inhalation of nitric oxide returns the pulmonary artery pressure to normal
C. Use of the prone position always results in improved oxygenation
D. Inhaled nitric oxide reduces mortality
E. PEEP requirement usually decreases during the fibroproliferatve phase.

QUESTION 88

In a patient with a cardiac pacemaker in place who requires an anaesthetic

A. The fourth letter defines functions for use in tachycardic episodes
B. Modern pacemaker function is not affected by volatile anaesthetic agents
C. VOO mode means function is more likely to be impaired by R on T induction of VF
D. Hyperkalaemia alters the threshold for capture
E. An increase in sympathetic tone may increase the paced rate

QUESTION 89

Omeprazole has important pharmacokinetic interactions with the following drugs

A. Phenytoin
B. Digoxin
C. Warfarin
D. Diazepam
E. Tetracycline

QUESTION 90

When interpreting pressures from the pulmonary artery catheter

A. PCWP greater than the pulmonary artery end diastolic pressure suggests incorrect catheter placement
B. PEEP causes an increase in pulmonary capillary wedge pressure
C. When using PEEP it is recommended that the ventilator be disconnected to make measurements
D. Left atrial pressure reflects left ventricular end diastolic pressure in mitral stenosis
E. Tachycardia does not affect pulmonary capillary wedge pressure readings

Exam 4: Answers

ANSWER 1

A. FALSE   **B. TRUE**   **C. FALSE**   **D. FALSE**   **E. TRUE**

Normal body function depends upon a relatively constant body temperature. Thermoregulatory control occurs in the hypothalamus. Responses activated by cold are controlled from the posterior hypothalamus while those activated by warmth are controlled primarily from the anterior hypothalamus. Stimulation of the anterior hypothalamus causes cutaneous vasodilatation and sweating. Posterior hypothalamic stimulation results in shivering and cutaneous vasoconstriction. Body heat is lost primarily by radiation and conduction (70%), with sweat vaporization accounting for 27% of heat loss, respiration 2%, and 1% via urine and faeces. As part of the endocrine response to cold there is increased catecholamine secretion and an increased secretion of TSH. Interleukin-1, produced by monocytes, macrophages, and Kupffer cells often as a result of endotoxin, has widespread effects in the body which includes fever production. This may be due to local release of prostaglandins into the hypothalamus stimulating fever as it is known that the anti-pyretic effect of aspirin is exerted directly on the hypothalamus, and aspirin also inhibits prostaglandin synthesis.

Ref: Ganong. Review of Medical Physiology. Appleton & Lane. 16th Ed. Ch 14. pg 225-230. Temperature regulation.

ANSWER 2

A. FALSE   **B. TRUE**   **C. FALSE**   **D. TRUE**   **E. FALSE**

The estimated nutritional reserves of a 70 kg man are:-

Carbohydrate	- 0.2 kg, mainly liver glycogen
Protein	- 4-6 kg, mainly as muscle
Fat	- 12-15 kg, mainly as adipose triglycerides

Average daily nutritional demands are:-

35 - 40 kcal/kg (145 - 170 kJ/kg) = 2450 - 2800 kcal (10,150 - 11,900 kJ)

Nitrogen intake of 0.2g/kg = 14 gm

Calorie:nitrogen ratio of 180:1

In hypercatabolic patients a lower caloric input of 30 kcal/kg/24 hrs with a lower calorie:nitrogen ratio, 80:1 or less, has been advocated.

Ref: T.E. OH.Intensive Care Manual. Butterworths. 3rd Edition. Ch 81. Enteral Nutrition

ANSWER 3

A. TRUE   B. FALSE   C. FALSE   D. TRUE   E. FALSE

In aortic stenosis the normal aortic valve area decreases from 3 cm^2 to less than 1cm^2. Without increased left ventricular systolic pressures the blood flow across the valve is dependent on the pressure gradient. With compensatory hypertrophy of the left ventricle the aortic valve gradient will increase. However later in the disease as the left ventricle dilates and further fails the left ventricular valve gradient will fall as cardiac output falls. A relatively slower heart rate is important to allow adequate time for left ventricular filling and emptying. The increased impedance to left ventricular emptying is at valve level and so changes in systemic vascular resistance will not signicantly affect left ventricular emptying. However a decrease in systemic vascular resistance may lead to critical reductions in myocardial perfusion. Episodes of myocardial ischaemia should be treated by firstly increasing systemic perfusion pressure. Vasodilators such as nitrates should be used with extreme caution if at all.

Ref: Hensley. The practice of cardiac anaesthesia. Little, Brown. Anaesthetic management for the treatment of valvular heart disease.

ANSWER 4

A. TRUE   B. FALSE   C. FALSE   D. FALSE   E. TRUE

Doppler monitoring measures blood flow by assessing the change in the frequency of a signal reflected by the blood cells moving through the descending aorta. It cannot measure pressures, and left ventricular wall motion may be observed by trans-oesophageal echocardiography. Cardiac output measurement relies on a calculated aortic cross-sectional area, not on direct measurement. It has been validated by comparison with thermodilution.

ANSWER 5

A. TRUE   B. FALSE   C. FALSE   D. FALSE   E. FALSE

An ejection systolic murmer may be due to a valvular lesion or may be functional, innocent, and not related to a structural cardiac lesion. Antibiotic cover is recommended for patients with congenital heart disease or acquired valve disease receiving dental or operative treatment. 2D echocardiography will demonstrate calcification or valvular thickening and LVH secondary to aortic stenosis. Doppler echocardiography works out pressures from the velocity of blood within the heart and can be used to determine gradient across the valve. Values over 50 mmHg are considered significant, although a poor left ventricle may contract so weakly against a severely stenosed valve that a large gradient is not achieved. Goldmann noted no increase in peroperative mortality with mitral valve disease but a 13% mortality in patients with important aortic stenosis.

Ref: Kaufman L. Anaesthesia Review 10 (Butterworths). Ch1.

ANSWER 6

A. FALSE   B. FALSE   C. TRUE   D. TRUE   E. TRUE

MMA bleeding leads to extradurals which are usually unilateral and associated with skull fractures.

Ref: Yentis, Hirsch and Smith. Anaesthesia A-Z. Butterworths. pp 422

ANSWER   7

A. TRUE   B. TRUE   C. FALSE   D. TRUE   E. FALSE

Babies often lose up to 10% of their weight in the first few days of life. Their cardiac output is about 180 ml/kg. There has been great debate about the ability of neonates to perceive pain, EEG evidence would suggest that they can. However, great care must be taken when using opioids in pre-term babies up to 50-60 weeks post-conceptual age. Apnoeic episodes may occur after GA and are more likely when opioids are used. Non steroidal anti inflammatory drugs are not recommended for use in infants/neonates. By inhibiting prostaglandin function they may affect ductal closure and interfere with renal function. Paracetamol up to 80 mg/kg/day is a useful alternative.

Ref: Scurr, feldman and Soni. Scientific Foundations 4th ed. Heinemann. pp 518.

ANSWER   8

A. FALSE   B. TRUE   C. TRUE   D. FALSE   E. FALSE

Hypovolaemic shock is due to inadequate left ventricular preload, which usually requires a relative or absolute reduction in circulating blood volume of 15 - 25 %. Cellular ischaemia results in anaerobic metabolism with depletion of ATP and lactic acidosis. As shock progresses the sympathetic vasoconstriction is overcome by the accumulation of local tissue metabolites, capillary permeability increases resulting in the extravasation of plasma which further compounds the intravascular hypovolaemia. Hyperventilation occurs due to peripheral chemoreceptor stimulation and later by the metabolic acidosis. Both hepatic arterial and portal venous blood flow are reduced in shock.

Ref: T.E. OH. Intensive Care Manual. Butterworths. 3rd Ed. Ch 58. Hypovolaemic shock

ANSWER   9

A. TRUE   B. TRUE   C. FALSE   D. FALSE   E. TRUE

Torsade de pointes is a polymorphic ventricular tachycardia with a prolonged QT interval. It is important to recognise because anti-arrhythmic agents prolong the QT interval and may make the situation worse. The causes are:-

Bradycardia

Anti-arrhythmic agents, particularly quinidine and disopyramide

Congenital (Romano ward syndrome)

Hypokalaemia

Hypomagnesaemia

Tricyclics

Erythromycin

Ref: Current Anaesthesia and Critical Care 1995; Vol 6, No 3: pg155-161. Diagnosis and management of tachyarrhythmias

ANSWER   10

A. TRUE   B. FALSE   C. FALSE   D. FALSE   E. TRUE

Horners syndome is the triad of enopthalmos, ptosis and miosis. Nasal congestion and anhydrosis are common but ipsilateral. Remember that exomphalos is a neonatal condition!

Ref: Yentis, Hirsch, and Smith. Anaesthesia A-Z. Butterworths. pp 420

ANSWER 11

A. TRUE   B. TRUE   C. TRUE   D. TRUE   E. TRUE

Loss of iron from epithelial cells is responsible for many of the features of iron deficiency anaemia such as glossitis and brittle hair and nails. Koilonychia refers to spoon shaped nails.

Dysphagia and glossitis form part of the Plummer Vinson or Paterson Brown Kelly syndrome. Parotid gland enlargement is rare but can occur in severe iron deficiency anaemia.

Ref: Kumar & Clark. Clinical Medicine. Balliere Tindall. Ch 6

ANSWER 12

A. FALSE   B. TRUE   C. TRUE   D. FALSE   E. FALSE

Compartment syndrome occurs when the interstitial tissue pressure rises above that of the capillary bed. Local ischaemia to nerve and muscle results. It may be initiated by crush injuries and closed or open fractures. Arterial injuries are indicated by diminished pulses, bruits or thrills, pallor, coolness, decreased sensation, weakness and reduced capillary and venous filling. Calcaneal fractures are commonly caused by falls from height and may cause vertebral injury through transmission of force. Reimplantation of an amputated digit may be possible for up to 18 hours if it is cooled. Otherwise it is only viable for 6 hours. Injury to the distal median nerve will lead to loss of sensation in the index finger and inability of thenar contraction and thumb opposition.

Ref. Advanced Trauma Life Support Student Manual. American College of Surgeons.

ANSWER 13

A. FALSE   B. TRUE   C. FALSE   D. FALSE   E. FALSE

Neurolept malignant syndrome is an idiosyncratic reaction to drugs (phenothiazines, thioxanthines, amantadine, lithium, butyrophenones and tricyclic antidepressants). It is a central disorder in association with a peripheral muscular mechanism and therefore differs from MH which is entirely peripheral. Features include the slow onset of muscle rigidity, akinesia, tremor and extrapyramidal movement abnormalities. A temperature of >39°C is usual, and variations in conscious level and autonomic function are not uncommon. Rhabdomyolysis, myoglobinuria, renal failure, leucocytosis and abnormal liver function may occur. The offending drug should be withdrawn, and rehydration and cooling commenced. Dantrolene and bromocriptine have been used successfully. ICU management is often required. Airway control, ventilation and circulatory stability should be achieved.

Ref: Hillman and Bishop. Clinical Intensive Care. Cambridge University Press. Ch 12.

ANSWER 14

A. TRUE   B. TRUE   C. FALSE   D. TRUE   E. TRUE

The Michaelis Menten equation describes how an enzymatically controlled reaction occurs at a speed determined by the concentration of enzyme and concentration of substrate. Receptor proteins in cell membranes often attach to G-proteins composed of 3 sub-units. Of these sub-units the alpha unit can be released on stimulation of the receptor, and then G-protein, to affect enzymes (including cAMP and cGMP), open ion channels, or cause gene transcription. A variety of intracellular compounds act as enzymatic second messengers for compounds or electric events which stimulate cells. Cyclic AMP is the messenger via which a variety of hormones function; these include ACTH, TSH, vasopressin, glucagon and the catecholamines.

Calcium ions entering a cell can stimulate calmodulin which can have a variety of effects including activating myosin kinase to produce smooth muscle contraction.

Ref: Guyton and Hall. Textbook of Medical Physiology. Chapter 69. Protein metabolism. Chapter 16. The microcirculation and lymphatic system. Chapter 68 Lipid metabolism.

ANSWER   15

A. FALSE   B. TRUE   C. TRUE   D. FALSE   E. FALSE

Duodenal perforation is ten times more common than gastric ulcer perforation. Leakage of fluid into the para-colic gutter may produce clinical findings resembling acute appendicitis. A moderate rise in serum amylase may occur in duodenal perforation. In approximately 65% of cases there is free gas beneath the diaphragm on erect chest X-ray but absence does not exclude the diagnosis. This may be because the perforation can occur into the lesser sac or is rapidly sealed by omentum. In such cases a gastrograffin swallow should be performed.

Ref: Forrest, Carter, MacLeod. Principles and Practise of Surgery. Churchill Livingstone.

ANSWER   16

A. TRUE   B. TRUE   C. FALSE   D. FALSE   E. TRUE

Cyanosis occurs in Fallots because of the reversal of the normal left to right flow through the VSD by right ventricular obstruction and pulmonary stenosis. In transposition of the great arteries, cyanosis is a result of right ventricular blood ejected directly into the ascending aorta and left ventricular blood into the pulmonary artery. In coarctation, there is no right to left shunt.

In totally anomalous pulmonary venous drainage, a right to left shunt occurs through the atrial septum in order to maintain systemic flow when all the pulmonary veins drain into the right atrium or major systemic vein.

Ref: Weaherall, Ledingham & Warrell. Oxford Textbook of Medicine. vol 2 section 13

ANSWER   17

A. FALSE   B. FALSE   C. TRUE   D. TRUE   E. TRUE

The spleen is most commonly injured by blunt abdominal trauma. Splenectomy is reserved for those with uncontrolled haemorrhage, pulverised spleen or in those where time taken to repair the spleen may compromise survival. Partial splenic resection or use of local clotting substances (eg gelfoam) is an alternative to splenectomy. Peritoneal lavage is more sensitive than computerised tomography in detecting intra-peritoneal blood. In blunt trauma > 10000 red cells / mm3 of peritoneal fluid is a positive finding and can be used in most cases as the sole diagnostic test indicating laparotomy. Road traffic accidents account for most cases of blunt abdominal trauma. This may be associated with the use of seat belts.

Ref: Oh. Intensive Care Manual. Butterworths.

ANSWER   18

A. TRUE   B. TRUE   C. TRUE   D. TRUE   E. FALSE

Abrupt abdominal aortic cross-clamping causes a 15-35% reduction in stroke volume and cardiac output, coupled with an increased arterial blood pressure and up to 40% increase in systemic vascular resistance. Diminished venous return is due to the exclusion of blood flow to the pelvis and lower extremities and possibly due to redistribution of blood from the inferior to the superior vena cava.

Ref: Barash, Cullen and Stoelting. Clinical Anaesthesia. J.B. Lippincott Co.

ANSWER 19

A. FALSE   B. TRUE   C. TRUE   D. FALSE   E. TRUE

Equivalent doses of steroids are: hydrocortisone (20), cortisone (25), prednisolone (5), methylprednisolone (4), betamethasone (0.6) and dexamethasone (0.75). Mineralocorticoid/sodium retaining activity is greatest with hydrocortisone and cortisone, lesser with prednisolone, and least with methylprednisolone, betamethasone and dexamethasone.

Ref: Oh T. Intensive Care Manual (Butterworths) Ch45.

ANSWER 20

A. TRUE   B. TRUE   C. TRUE   D. TRUE   E. TRUE

Post gastrectomy syndromes include bilious vomiting, dumping and post-vagotomy diarrhoea. Hyperglycaemia may follow rapid gastric emptying (early dumping) and this is responsible for an increased insulin release which in turn may cause a reactive hypoglycaemia (late dumping). Vasomotor disturbances such as flushing, sweating and tachycardia are associated with dumping. Intestinal obstruction may result from adhesions post-gastrectomy.

Ref: Dunn & Rawlinson. Surgical Diagnosis and Management. Blackwell Scientific Publishers.

ANSWER 21

A. TRUE   B. FALSE   C. FALSE   D. TRUE   E. TRUE

Methyl dopa competes as a substrate with dopa and is converted into the false neurotransmitter alpha methylnoradrenaline. This causes inhibition of sympathetic outflow and a reduction in systemic vascular resistance. Adverse effects include allergy, sedation, headache, nightmares, depression, constipation and a positive Coombs test. Gynaecomastia and lactation can occur and are due to removal of the supresion of prolactin secretion usually caused by dopamine.

Ref: Laurence and Bennett. Clinical Pharmacology (Fifth Edition) Churchill Livingstone. Ch 21.

ANSWER 22

A. TRUE   B. FALSE   C. FALSE   D. TRUE   E. FALSE

Aminophylline therapeutic range = 10-20 mg/l (toxic at 20 mg/l)

Diazepam therapeutic range = 0.5-2.5 mcg/l (lethal at 50 mcg/l)

Digoxin therapeutic range = 1-2 mcg/l (toxic > 2mcg/l)

Phenytoin therapeutic range = 8-20 mg/l (toxic at 30 mg/l)

Lignocaine is toxic at 6 mg/l

Ref: OH T. Intensive Care Manual (Butterworths) Appendix 5

ANSWER   23

A. FALSE   B. TRUE   C. TRUE   D. TRUE   E. TRUE

Myocardial blood flow is tightly linked to metabolic need or O_2 demand. Oxygen extraction is normally 70% so increased O_2 demand cannot be met by increased extraction except to a small degree and is therefore met by increased flow. Free fatty acids and glucose are normally the prime energy source but during exercise lactate takes on a more significant role. Collaterals in humans do develop in the sub-endocardium although they are not normal arteries in structure or nature and possess increased resistance to flow. A variety of vasodilatory and contrictor influences apply - both neural and humoral. Of the latter nitric oxide and endothelins are among the most potent.

Ref: Priebe & Skarvan. Cardiovascular Physiology. BMJ Publishing. Chapter 4. Coronary Physiology.

ANSWER   24

A. FALSE   B. TRUE   C. FALSE   D. TRUE   E. TRUE

Train of four = 4 supramaximal stimuli at 2Hz with a fixed pulse width of 0.2 ms. Force of contraction continues to slightly increase above the supramaximal threshold as a result of direct muscle stimulation. Therefore delivered current should ideally be 10-20% above the threshold. A train of four stimuli is used to detect fade on repetitive stimulation following non-depolarizing blockade. Fade is due to to non-depolarizer blockade of pre-junctional ACh receptors (which maintain ACH output with repetitive nerve stimulation). Post tetanic facilitation enables a response to occur when none was detectable following single twitches or TO4. The post tetanic count consists of a 5s 50Hz stimulus followed by a 3s pause and then single twitches at 1Hz. The number of detectable twitches is inversely related to intensity of block. Double burst stimulation = 3 x 50Hz stimuli separated by 0.75s.

ANSWER   25

A. FALSE   B. FALSE   C. TRUE   D. FALSE   E. FALSE

In COPD there is inflammation of the small airways and destruction of the lung parenchyma. The latter leads to a reduction in elastic recoil, the former to a reduction in airway patency. In order to keep the same ventilation when there is expiratory airflow obstruction, these patients breathe with a higher respiratory rate and a lower tidal volume. The airflow limitation, hyper-inflation, respiratory acidosis, and hypophosphataemia sometimes present result in an increased propensity to respiratory muscle fatigue. As alveoli may empty slowly during positive pressure ventilation, inspiration may commence before expiration is complete. This gas trapping leads to the development of auto-PEEP and alveolar overdistension with its attendant risks. High carbohydrate diets tend to increase $PaCO_2$ due to the higher R/Q than high fat diets, but there is little evidence to show a difference in outcome using fatty diets. Achieving normal blood gases may increase the chance of ventilator induced lung injury and many centres accept some degree of hypoxia and respiratory acidosis.

Ref: Aubier M. Pathophysiology and therapy of chronic obstructive pulmonary disease. Current Opinion in Critical Care 1995;1:11-15

ANSWER 26

A. FALSE   B. TRUE   C. FALSE   D. TRUE   E. FALSE

Serum amylase levels do not correlate with severity or mortality. Mumps, Epstein Barr virus, mycoplasma, hepatitis and ascariasis can all cause pancreatitis. 25% of patients have hypocalcaemia due to concomitant hypoproteinaemia and intraperitoneal saponification of calcium. Total parenteral nutrition is indicated for nutritional support as patients should be "nil by mouth", it does not however reduce the glands enzyme content.

Ref: Oh. Intensive Care Manual. 3rd edition. Butterworths. Part III.

ANSWER 27

A. FALSE   B. FALSE   C. TRUE   D. TRUE   E. TRUE

Most patients with gastric ulcers have normal or low acid outputs whereas most with duodenal ulcer secrete excess acid and pepsinogen. Though the relationship between pain and food is variable, those with duodenal ulcer typically complain of pain when they are hungry. Ranitidine is an H_2 receptor antagonist. It is more successful in the treatment of duodenal ulcer because it can reduce acid secretion by 60% over 24 hours and most duodenal ulcers are associated with a raised acid secretion. Because of its relative lack of side effects it is still used in the treatment of gastric ulcer. Constipation is a side effect of treatment with aluminium salts whereas diarrhoea occurs with magnesium salts. Hyperparathyroidism raises serum calcium which stimulates acid secretion.

Ref: Kumar & Clark. Clinical Medicine. Balliere Tindall. Ch 4

ANSWER 28

A. TRUE   B. FALSE   C. TRUE   D. FALSE   E. TRUE

Pyloric stenosis occurs in 1/300 births. Vomiting produces defects of water, H^+, Na^+, Cl^- and K^+. Any hyponatraemia occurs later when Na^+ is lost to accompany HCO3- in urine. A neonate can only concentrate urine to 500-700 mOsm/l and the urine will possibly show a paradoxical acid state due to H^+ loss. Hypochloraemia is due to gastric losses of Cl^-.

Ref: Stehling L. Common problems in pediatric anesthesia. Chapter 13.

ANSWER 29

A. TRUE   B. FALSE   C. FALSE   D. FALSE   E. TRUE

End tidal PCO_2 will rise as a result of hypoventilation, CO_2 inflation during laparoscopy, inadequate fresh gas flow, exhausted soda lime and hyperthermia. Hypotension and air embolism will both cause a fall in end tidal CO_2 and airway obstruction will prevent any reading.

Ref: Miller RD. Anesthesia 4th ed. Churchill Livingstone. Ch 17

ANSWER 30

A. FALSE   B. TRUE   C. FALSE   D. FALSE   E. TRUE

A high anion gap acidosis occurs when an unmeasured anion is responsible for the acidosis, and serum chloride is lower than would be expected from serum electrolytes and bicarbonate. The normal anion gap is 14 –18 mmol/l and mainly represents the unmeasured net negative charge on plasma proteins and can be estimated by:

Anion gap = ([Na] + [K]) - ([Cl] + [HCO3])

Normal anion gap acidoses are caused by increased bicarbonate loss from either the gut, e.g. ileostomy, or in the kidney, e.g. proximal tubular damage, decreased hydrogen ion secretion as ammonium e.g. distal renal tubular acidosis, or increased generation of HCl.

High anion gap acidoses are caused by accumulation of unmeasured acid. Organic acids such as hydroxybutyric and acetoacetic acids accumulate in diabetic ketoacidosis, inherited diseases with defective gluconeogenesis or pyruvate oxidation such as G-6-PD deficiency result in the accumulation of lactic acid as does tissue hypoxia. Exogenous acids such as salicylic acid and the ingestion of ethanol, methanol, fructose, sorbitol and metformin can all elevate the anion gap. Botulism results in a respiratory acidosis as a result of hypoventilation.

Ref: Current Anaesthesia and Critical Care 1996; Vol 7, No 4: pg176-181. Physiology and pathophysiology of fluids and electrolytes.

ANSWER   31

A. TRUE   B. FALSE   C. FALSE   D. TRUE   E. FALSE

The patient giving consent for a procedure in England must be over the age of 16 and of sound mind, ie unaffected by premedicant drugs. Verbal consent is valid, but ought to be witnessed. Consent may also be implied or expressed (eg by allowing insertion of a cannula, the patient is demonstrating consent without actually expressing it). Emergency life-saving surgery can proceed without consent where unobtainable, provided an average reasonable adult would agree to the procedure. Consent in mental illness may be given by the closest relative or an officer of the appropriate institution, rarely by the courts.

Ref: Yentis Hirsch and Smith. Anaesthesia A to Z. Butterworth Heinemann.

ANSWER   32

A. FALSE   B. FALSE   C. TRUE   D. TRUE   E. FALSE

Sevoflurane is a fluorinated ether related structurally to isoflurane. However, isoflurane is an isomer of enflurane. The excitatory phenomena seen when rapidly increasing the inspired concentration of desflurane are not observed with sevoflurane. Intracranial pressure increases at high inspired concentrations of sevoflurane; even at 0.5-1 MAC there is a minimal effect. Although the amount of compound A that is produced during a variety of clinical scenarios is less than that shown to be toxic to animals, the degradation of sevoflurane is temperature dependent. Free fluoride concentration increases during sevoflurane anaesthesia and may exceed 50 micromol/l in some circumstances.

Ref: Smith I, Nathanson M, White PF. Sevoflurane- a long-awaited volatile anaesthetic. British Journal of Anaesthesia 1996;76:435-445

ANSWER   33

A. TRUE   B. FALSE   C. TRUE   D. TRUE   E. FALSE

MRI relies on the radiofrequency radiation emitted by an unpaired electron exposed to pulses of radiofrequency radiation. Examples of atoms with unpaired electrons include H-1, P-31, F-

19 & C-13. Neither C-12 or H-2 have unpaired electrons. MRI is the technique of choice to image the posterior fossa of the skull. MRI scanners have a marked line at which the field falls to between 5 and 50 Gauss. Infusion devices are not affected until the field reaches 100 Gauss.

Ref: Blunt, M.C. and Urquhart, J.C. (1997) The Anaesthesia Viva: Physics, Measurement, Clinical Anaesthesia, Anatomy and Safety, London: Greenwich Medical Media.

ANSWER 34
A. FALSE   B. FALSE   C. FALSE   D. TRUE   E. FALSE

Status epilepticus is defined as the occurrence of seizures that persist for longer than 30 minutes or lack of recovery between each fit. The brain is at risk from cerebral oedema, hypoxia and neuronal damage. It has a mortality of 3-20%. The causes are varied but include drug overdose or withdrawal, metabolic disorders (hypoglycaemia and electrolyte imbalances must always be excluded), ischaemia, head injury, infection/pyrexia, intracerebral tumour, eclampsia and underlying, inadequately controlled epilepsy. Treatment should be aimed at maintaining a protected airway and stopping the fits whilst excluding any reversible causes. Diazepam is usually the first line medication, with phenytoin added in if fits recur or are felt a high risk. Paraldehyde PR is useful in children and clonazepam or diazepam infusions can also be used at this stage if cardiorespiratory function is monitored. If seizures still occur, thiopentone infusion is required, necessitating endotracheal intubation and assisted ventilation. There are no particular features of epilepsy that contraindicate the use of atracurium but paralysis, although useful if hyperthermia or rhabdomyolysis are present, will mask the seizures.

Ref: Hillman and Bishop. Clinical Intensive Care. Cambridge University Press. Ch 25. Advanced Life Support Group. Advanced Paediatric Life Support; The Practical Approach. BMJ. CH 11.

ANSWER 35
A. FALSE   B. TRUE   C. TRUE   D. TRUE   E. FALSE

MUGA involves the use of technetium-99 labelled red cells. It is used to determine peak systolic volume in relation to diastolic volume and can detect regional wall motion abnormalities. This is achieved by collecting a series of counts with a gamma camera which have been time marked against the ECG complexes, it thus requires a regular cardiac rhythm. Counts from epochs of 30-50 ms within each cardiac cycle are summated over a period of time to give an overall picture of cardiac function. Preoperative ejection fraction of <35% by MUGA has been shown to correlate with early perioperative infarction (Pasternack).

Myocardial perfusion may be assessed using the potassium analogue thallium-201. It is injected into a vein and is taken up by myocytes in proportion to the perfusion and viability of the cell. Stress can be induced by exercise or administration of dobutamine. Ischaemia may be provoked using dipyridamole or adenosine which create steal by vasodilatation of normal circulation. Reversibility of a perfusion defect demonstrates a non-infarcted area that may benefit from grafting.

Ref: Kaufman L. Anaesthesia Review 10. (Churchill Livingstone) Ch1.

ANSWER 36
A. FALSE   B. TRUE   C. FALSE   D. TRUE   E. FALSE

Pulse oximetry is based on the Beer-Lambert Law of light transmission (Hoppe-Seyler recognised in 1864 that the absorbance of blue and green light was due to haemoglobin, and that it varied with the aeration of the blood). Oximetry is accurate to 2% at best, but sudden falls in

SaO_2 show delayed falls in SpO_2. Despite oximetry alerting anaesthetists to the presence of hypoxia, and reducing the incidence of intraoperative myocardial ischaemia, there is no evidence that its use reduces the incidence of post-operative complications.

Ref: Paulus, D.A. (1993) Noninvasive Monitoring of Oxygen and Carbon Dioxide. In: Carlson, R.W. and Geheb, M.A. (Eds.) Principles and Practice of Medical Intensive Care, pp. 203-220. Philadelphia: W B Saunders

ANSWER 37

A. TRUE B. TRUE C. TRUE D. TRUE E. FALSE

Portal hypertension occurs when the portal venous pressure exceeds 10mmHg. Causes are divided into pre-hepatic (20%) eg. portal vein thrombosis, hepatic (80%) eg. cirrhosis and post-hepatic (rare) eg.tricuspid incompetence and Budd-Chiari syndrome (hepatic vein thrombosis). It causes dilatation of porta-systemic collaterals (hence oesophageal varices, gastric venous dilation and rectal varices) including the epidural veins hence extradural blockade is contraindicated. Hypoalbuminaemia and ascites, splenomegaly and thrombocytopaenia all occur, along with encephalopathy.

Ref: McLatchie. Oxford Handbook of Clinical Surgery. Oxford University Press.

ANSWER 38

A. TRUE B. FALSE C. TRUE D. FALSE E. FALSE

The stress response to surgery is complex and is modified by anaesthesia preoperatively, intra-operatively and in the recovery stage. Considering opioids, morphine 2-4 mg/kg and fentanyl 50-200 mcg/kg will abolish the stress response to major surgery. Sympathetic nervous stimulation plays a part in the stress response but a number of hormones are released, including TSH, FSH, ADH etc. Mechanical ventilation increases the levels of ADH and decreases free water excretion. PEEP causes higher rises in noradrenaline.

Ref: Scurr, Feldman and Soni. Scientific Foundations 4th ed. Heineman. pp 354-357

ANSWER 39

A. FALSE B. TRUE C. TRUE D. FALSE E. TRUE

Gastric tonometry estimates the gastric intramucosal pH and therefore it has been suggested that it is a technique that will provide early detection of splanchnic ischaemia in the critically ill.

The technique involves introducing a small, fixed volume of saline (or perhaps gelatin) into a silicon balloon in the gastric lumen. Equilibration occurs and the PCO_2 of the saline after a set period is converted into the luminal PCO_2 by a correction factor (dependent on the equilibration time to acknowledge incomplete equilibration will have taken place). This luminal PCO_2, if produced by luminal cell respiration, is the intracellular PCO_2. This is then entered into a modified Henderson-Hasselbalch equation;

$$pHi = 6.1 + \log [(HCO_3) / (PCO_2 \times 0.003)]$$

where HCO_3 is the measurement of arterial bicarbonate (which is suggested to be the same as intramucosal bicarbonate). A value of 7.32 or less is outside 2 standard deviations of the mean of healthy individuals and therefore thought to be abnormal. Several inaccuracies can occur including air in the sample, inadequate equilibration, a source of intraluminal CO_2 (food in the stomach). Ranitidine therefore increases the reproducibility of results in those capable of producing gastric acid. pHi predicts morbidity and mortality in perioperative and critically ill patients. However, assumptions that are made during the calculation (with some arguing that it only reflects systemic acidosis) and the inaccuracies that occur without very close attention to detail make many suspect its usefulness.

Ref: Sutcliffe NP, Mostafa SM. pHi: a review of the literature. Clinical Intensive Care 1996;7:258-264

ANSWER 40

A. TRUE   B. FALSE   C. TRUE   D. FALSE   E. TRUE

Tramadol is a racemic mixture of (+)tramadol and (-)tramadol and is an analgesic with a potency 5-10 times less than morphine. It has a preferential effect at mu opioid receptors and it also inhibits noradrenaline and 5-HT neuronal reuptake. It is thought that all these actions play a part in its centrally mediated analgesic effect and explains why, in volunteer studies, only 30% of its analgesic effects could be reversed by naloxone. It is not associated with significant respiratory depression and has low abuse, dependence and tolerance potential. However, it is not licensed for intraoperative use due to a high incidence of awareness (that may be due to the minimal sedative effect of the drug) It also causes postoperative nausea (incidence of 30-35%) and also may cause dizziness, dry mouth, sweating, headache and mild hypertension.

Ref: Eggers K, Power I. Tramadol. British Journal of Anaesthesia 1995;74:247-249

ANSWER 41

A. TRUE   B. FALSE   C. TRUE   D. FALSE   E. FALSE

Nitric oxide is a widespread biological mediator. It is one of the (and may be the only) endothelial derived relaxing factor. It is synthesised from L-arginine by the action of nitric oxide synthases, of which there are endothelial, neuronal and inducible types. L-citrulline is a product of its synthesis, which can be increased by administering L-arginine, and reduced by administering an L-arginine analogue e.g. N-monomethyl-L-arginine (L-NMMA). It is a free radical and diffuses into cells where it activates guanylate cyclase. Cyclic GMP levels therefore rise and cause vascular dilatation. This is the final common pathway through which all the nitrovasodilators work. Other actions include inhibition of platelet aggregation, neuronal communication, host defence response and perhaps inhibition of uterine contraction.

When inhaled in the acute lung injury, hypoxia and pulmonary hypertension may be reduced. The minimum effective dose should be given. Monitoring of inspired and local nitric oxide and nitrogen dioxide (a cytotoxic metabolite) concentrations, methaemoglobin levels and haemorrhagic occurrences must be carried out. Nitric oxide is not licensed for this indication.

Ref: Vallance P, Collier J. Biology and clinical relevance of nitric oxide. British Medical Journal 1994;309:453-457

ANSWER 42

A. TRUE   B. FALSE   C. FALSE   D. TRUE   E. TRUE

Chronic pancreatitis is commoner in men than in women, and is especially associated with alcohol abuse. Other causes include obstruction of the ampulla of Vater by calculus or tumour, post-traumatic, cystic fibrosis, hyperparathyroidism and primary sclerosing cholangitis. Chronic pancreatitis presents with abdominal pain, weight loss, steatorrhea, malabsorption and glucose intolerance. It is rarely fatal.

Ref: McLatchie. Oxford Handbook of Clinical Surgery. Oxford University Press.

ANSWER 43

A. FALSE   B. TRUE   C. TRUE   D. FALSE   E. TRUE

The maximum arterial PO_2 that can be achieved without hyperbaric therapy is 90kPa and can be calculated from the alveolar gas equation in healthy volunteers breathing 100% oxygen. The relationship between arterial and tissue PO_2 varies from tissue to tissue and can be limited by oxygen mediated vasoconstriction in organs such as the brain. Once 5 atmospheres has been reached whole body oyxgen requirements can be met by the oxygen dissolved in blood. The use of hyperbaric oyxgen therapy has waned and is now mainly used for carbon monoxide poisoning and anaerobic infections.

ANSWER 44

A. TRUE   B. FALSE   C. FALSE   D. FALSE   E. TRUE

The mainstream capnograph consists of a carbon dioxide measuring adaptor placed in the circuit. The sidestream capnograph suctions gas from the breathing circuit into a cell. Both measure carbon dioxide by infra-red light absorption. The mainstream analyser can cause traction on the endotracheal tube and its radiant heat generation can cause burns. This is less of a problem with newer models. However the sidestream analyser requires a sample of the fresh gas flow to operate. High aspiration rates (250 ml / min) and low dead space apparatus increase sensitivity but may entrain fresh gas from the circuit causing dilution. Low aspiration rate (50 ml / min) types are less sensitive and can underestimate carbon dioxide levels during rapid breathing. Sidestream analysers require water traps as precipitation can occur in the aspiration tube and cause obstruction. Capnography does not reliably detect endobronchial intubation.

Ref: Morgan, Mikhail. Clinical Anesthesiology. 2nd Edition. Prentice Hall International Inc.

ANSWER 45

A. TRUE   B. FALSE   C. TRUE   D. FALSE   E. FALSE

The majority of poisonings can be adequately managed with supportive care alone. Specific treatment with antidotes is required in only a small proprtion of cases, but may be life saving. Ethanol is the antidote for ethylene glycol, as well as methanol, poisoning. Pralidoxime, along with atropine, is the antidote for organophosphate poisoning. While propranolol can be used to control the tachycardia, hypokalaemia and hyperglycaemia associated with theophylline poisoning it is not a specific antidote. Remember that flumazenil does not have a product licence for the reversal of benzodiazepine overdose as it can precipitate convulsions in patients who are dependent on benzodiazepines or in those who have also ingested a drug which can cause convulsions in overdose eg tricyclics or theophylline.

Ref: Current Anaesthesia and Critical Care 1996. Vol 7, No 2: pg 95-100. Concepts in the management of poisoning.

ANSWER 46

A. FALSE   B. TRUE   C. TRUE   D. TRUE   E. TRUE

Due to the poor survival of patients with established ARF and the high cost of treatment, various protocols have been developed to prevent ARF developing. The best time to protect the kidney from an insult is before it happens and it is therefore useful to identify the groups of patients at high risk of developing ARF. Recognised risk factors for developing ARF include:- Old age, Diabetes, Arterial disease, Pre-existing renal impairment, Myeloma, Nephrotic syndrome, Chronic liver disease, Obstructive jaundice.

Ref: British Journal of Hospital Medicine 1996; Vol 55, No 4: pg 162-166. Prevention of acute renal failure.

ANSWER 47

A. TRUE   B. TRUE   C. FALSE   D. TRUE   E. FALSE

Respiratory causes of clubbing:

bronchial carcinoma (esp. squamous cell), chronic suppurative lung disease eg bronchiectasis, abscess, empyema, pulmonary fibrosis eg cryptogenic fibrosing alveolitis, pleural and mediastinal tumours eg mesothelioma.

Cardiovascular causes:

cyanotic heart disease, subacute bacterial endocarditis- not in acute endocarditis as it takes months to develop. Hence it is not seen in neonates with cyanotic heart disease till later.

Miscellaneous causes:

congenital, cirrhosis, inflammatory bowel disease

Ref: Kumar & Clark. Clinical Medicine. Balliere Tindall. Chapter 12.

ANSWER 48

A. TRUE   B. TRUE   C. FALSE   D. FALSE   E. TRUE

Most intravenous anaesthetic agents cause vasodilatation and/or depression of myocardial function. In shocked patients the central volume of distribution is decreased and this can result in relative overdosage of drugs resulting in hypotension and aggravation of any existing haemorrhagic shock. Reduced pulmonary perfusion decreases the uptake of volatile anaesthetic agents. Narcotic analgesics decrease sympathetic tone and may aggravate shock. Narcotics also cause respiratory depression, decrease intestinal motility and increase the incidence of nausea and vomiting. Narcotics should not be administered to spontaneously breathing head injured patients due to the risk of respiratory depression and subsequent rise in intracranial pressure. In trauma patients lower doses of anaesthetic agents are often utilised due to the fear or concern of hypotension and special attention must be paid to the problem of awareness as in one study the incidence was as high as 43%.

Ref: Current Anaesthesia and Critical Care. Churchill Livingstone. 1996. Vol 7, No 3, pg 125-138. Anaesthetic management of the trauma patient in the operating theatre.

ANSWER 49

A. FALSE   B. TRUE   C. TRUE   D. FALSE   E. FALSE

Surgical blood loss has not been shown to be significantly different whether hypotension is produced by vasodilatation or reduction in cardiac output. Na nitroprusside along with other vasodilators may produce rises in intracranial pressure at doses which produce moderate decreases in blood pressure. Mild coronary stenoses in some models do not lead to myocardial ischaemia in the face of hypotension although more severe stenoses will do so. Dead space will not necessarily rise if circulating volume is maintained but it will not be reduced.

Ref: Miller. Anesthesia. Deliberate Hypotension.

ANSWER 50

A. TRUE   B. FALSE   C. FALSE   D. TRUE   E. FALSE

This degree of blood loss represents 20% of this child's circulating volume which would be expected to be 1750 ml based on 70 ml/Kg. The physiological effects of blood loss in children differ from those in adults and are:-

LOSS < 25% OF CIRCULATING VOLUME

    Increased heart rate, normal blood pressure.

    Cool, clammy skin, collapsed veins

    Lethargic, irritable, combative

    Slightly decreased urine output

LOSS = 25% OF CIRCULATING VOLUME

    Increased heart rate, blood pressure normal or slightly reduced

    Cold, blotchy skin, peripheral cyanosis

    Dulled response to pain

    Significantly reduced urine output

LOSS > 25% OF CIRCULATING VOLUME

    Increased heart rate, thready pulse, reduced blood pressure

    Pale, cold, blotchy skin

    Often comatose

    Anuria

Ref: Current Anaesthesia and Critical care 1996; Vol 7, No 3: pg 146-151. Paediatric trauma anaesthesia.

ANSWER 51

A. TRUE   B. TRUE   C. TRUE   D. FALSE   E. TRUE

Indirectly acting sympathomimetics like ephedrine are unlikely to increase blood pressure in patients taking drugs which alter neuronal storage, uptake, metabolism or release of neurotransmitters. Reserpine depletes neuronal granules of noradrenaline. Alpha-methyl dopa acts as a false transmitter. Phenoxybenzamine and propranolol block peripheral receptors and industrial doses of directly acting sympathomometics may be required to overcome their blockade. Clonidine works on central adrenergic receptors and the peripheral effect of indirectly acting sympathomimetics is not decreased, in fact smaller doses may be required due to receptor up regulation.

Ref: Miller. Anesthesia. Churchill Livingstone. 4th Ed, Ch 27

ANSWER 52

A. FALSE   B. TRUE   C. TRUE   D. TRUE   E. TRUE

Most modern flowmeters are variable area flowmeters of 'rotameter' (TM) or ball and tube construction. Their principle of function depends on pressure drop across the orifice between 'float' and the walls of its container. This pressure drop in turn depends on the density of the gas and on the size and length of the orifice. This does depend on both gas density and float length in a tapered tube. Back pressure causes inaccuracy due to increase in gas density and static electricity is a particular problem especially in a dry climate.

Ref: Ward. Anaesthetic equipment. Chapter 8. The supply of anaesthetic gases.

ANSWER   53

A. TRUE   B. TRUE   C. TRUE   D. FALSE   E. FALSE

Pagets disease raises alkaline phosphatase to levels greater than five times the upper limit of normal and is due to increased osteoblastic activity. The raised alkaline phosphatase in malignant disease maybe of bony or hepatic origin, with the presence of both primary and secondary tumours at these sites. A number of specific alkaline phosphatases secreted by tumour cells also exist. Osteoporosis does not raise alkaline phosphatase unless complicated by collapse or fracture of bone. The placenta is another source of the enzyme, and raised alkaline phosphatase levels can occur in pregnancy, especially in the last trimester. Myocardial infarction leads to raised aspartate transaminase, normally < 35 iu/l, not alkaline phosphatase.

Ref: Marshall. Clinical Chemistry. Lippincott Company. Ch 17

ANSWER   54

A. TRUE   B. TRUE   C. TRUE   D. TRUE   E. FALSE

Scleroderma leads to alveolar wall breakdown, honeycomb cavity formation and fibrosis. Radiotherapy gives rise to sharply delineated areas of fibrosis which take up the shape of the treatment fields. Berylliosis after inhalational exposure leads to a chemical pneumonitis causing fibrosis with progression to pulmonary hypertension and cor pulmonale. Organophosphorus compounds inactivate the body complement of cholinesterase and so cause weakness, vomiting, colicky abdominal pain, profuse sweating and hypersalivation. Bronchoconstriction with bronchial hypersecretion also occur. Prompt treatment is needed to prevent respiratory depression, coma and death.

Ref: Weatherall, Ledingham & Warrell. Oxford Textbook of Medicine. vol 2 section 15, 16

ANSWER   55

A. TRUE   B. FALSE   C. FALSE   D. FALSE   E. TRUE

Sterilisation removes all bacteria, fungi, spores and viruses, which disinfection does not necessarily achieve. Autoclaving is the use of steam at above atmospheric pressure, and therefore at above 100C, for the purpose of sterilisation. Prion particles may not be removed by sterilisation. Gamma irradiation can be used for the sterilisation of pvc articles. However, if ethylene oxide is used subsequently, ethylene chlorohydrin is produced which is highly toxic. Chlorhexidine will remove bacteria but not their spores and can support the growth of gram -ve organisms in aqueous solution.

Ref: Dorsch & Dorsch. Understanding anaesthetic equipment: Construction, Care and Complications. Chapter 15. Cleaning and Sterilization.

ANSWER   56

A. FALSE   B. TRUE   C. TRUE   D. FALSE   E. FALSE

All types of eye surgery can be performed under local anaesthesia . The following are considered contraindications: 90 mins or longer for op, infants or children, mental retardation, excessive anxiety, uncontrolled cough, and inability to lie flat.

Ref: Berry C. Regional anaesthesia for cataract surgery. Br J Hosp Med.1993,49,689-701.

ANSWER 57

A. TRUE   B. TRUE   C. FALSE   D. FALSE   E. FALSE

Sepsis and multiorgan failure are the leading causes of mortality in the ICU. The cytokine network is triggered resulting in vasodilatation (causing relative hypovolaemia), loss of body fluids by sequestration, perspiring etc. (causing absolute hypovolaemia), myocardial depression (although baroreceptor reflex response to the hypotension more often results in a noticeable hyperdynamic circulation), maldistribution of blood flow and a resulting tissue hypoxia. Intravenous fluid is always required to restore circulating volume. Acceptable crystalloids are those that contain extracellular ions in preponderance (normal saline). Dextrose containing fluids will be distributed across cell membranes and expand intracellular volume in preference. Only once circulating volume and oxygenation are restored should vasoactive or inotropic agents be considered to increase the perfusion pressure. If myocardial depression is present, an inotrope should be the first choice. If, however, the cardiac ouput is well maintained, careful titration of a vasopressor to increase blood pressure is appropriate. Invasive cardiovascular monitoring is useful, and many would insist on the use of data derived from a pulmonary artery catheter.

Ref: Spiijkstra JJ, Thijs LG. Methods of resuscitation in septic shock. International Journal of Intensive Care 1995;2:40-47

ANSWER 58

A. TRUE   B. TRUE   C. FALSE   D. FALSE   E. FALSE

Other cardiovascular features include pericarditis and conduction defects. Pulmonary fibrosis and costochondral disease in rhematoid arthritis lead to a restrictive respiratory pattern. Renal impairment may also be due to pyelonephritis or drug treatment eg penicillamine. Skin is easily damaged because it is atrophic.

Ref: Yentis, Hirsch & Smith. Anaesthesia A to Z. Butterworth Heinemann. p391.

ANSWER 59

A. TRUE   B. TRUE   C. TRUE   D. FALSE   E. TRUE

Although there is no anatomical lower oesophageal sphincter the lower 2-3 cms of oesophagus are intra-abdominal and the presence of of a functional flap valve at the lower end of the oesophagus help prevent gastric reflux. Ranitidine reaches peak levels at 1 hour and remains at effective plasma concentrations for 8 hours after oral dosing. The reflex rise in lower oesophageal pressure helps maintain a safe barrier pressure with modest rises in intragastric pressure.

Ref: Miller Anesthesia. Chapter 43. Pulmonary aspiration of gastric contents.

ANSWER 60

A. FALSE   B. TRUE   C. FALSE   D. TRUE   E. FALSE

AIDS is the clinical manifestation of infection by HIV viruses. Infection with HIV results in several immune defects, the most important being impaired cell mediated immunity due to a deficiency in CD4+ T-cells. Some patients have defective antibody-mediated responses, particularly in paediatric HIV infection. By definition AIDS results in a severe immunodeficiency resulting in 'major' opportunistic infections by protozoa, viruses, fungi, spirochaetes and mycobacteria. Recurrent bacterial infections only occur if there is concurrent antibody deficiency (B-cell function). While ventilation may be indicated in Pneumocystis pneumonia, it is unlikely to be of benefit if adequate anti-microbial therapy is already being given.

Ref: T.E. OH. Intensive Care Manual. Butterworths. 3rd Ed, Ch 62, Immunodeficiency.

ANSWER   61

A. TRUE   B. TRUE   C. TRUE   D. TRUE   E. FALSE

Visceral nociceptive afferents pass via the sympathetic ganglion to the dorsal horn of the spinal cord. The pain associated is diffuse, poorly localised and of a dull or vague nature, and is commonly associated with nausea and vomiting. It may be referred to the cutaneous area corresponding to that dorsal horn, and may be associated with allodynia and hyperalgesia over that area. The spinal cord levels of the viscera are frequently overlapping, so there is often difficulty in diagnosis, however the small intestine is T9–T10 and the urinary bladder T11–L2.

Ref: Cousins, M. (1994) Acute and post-operative pain. In: Wall, P.D. and Melzack, R. (Eds.) Textbook of Pain, 3rd edn. pp. 357-386. Edinburgh: Churchill Livingstone

ANSWER   62

A. FALSE   B. TRUE   C. FALSE   D. TRUE   E. FALSE

In a study which compared PCA with intrathecal opioids following caesarean section, superior analgesia was seen with intrathecal opioids but the differences in analgesia were minimal after the first 16 hours and also side effects were less frequent with PCA.

Whenever opioids are administered, respiratory depression and hypoxaemia is likely to occur and PCA is no exception. The overall incidence of severe respiratory depression associated with intravenous opioid use has been found to be 0.56%. However, breaking this down reveals the incidence of respiratory depression with continuous morphine infusions is 1.65%, PCA plus a background infusion is similar but with PCA alone the incidence is 0.27%.

In a large study examining the incidence of mishaps during 3299 PCA uses the overall incidence was 1.2%. The breakdown of these mishaps revealed that 36% were equipment malfunctions, 21% improper loading, 17% documentation errors, 14% programming errors and 14% adverse drug reactions.

Ref: Current Anaesthesia and Critical Care. Churchill Livingstone. 1995. Vol 6, No 2, pg 76 - 80. Patient-controlled analgesia

ANSWER   63

A. FALSE   B. FALSE   C. TRUE   D. TRUE   E. TRUE

Neisseria meningococcus is the commonest cause of bacterial meningitis in UK. An increasing proportion of meningococci have become sulphonamide resistant but all strains remain sensitive to penicillin. The CSF glucose is reduced to less than half of the blood value. Normal CSF protein is 0.1 - 0.4 g/l, in bacterial meningitis it is 0.5 - 2 g/l. Pericarditis is a septic or reactive complication of septicaemia especially with meningococcus. No vaccine is available for Group B meningococcus (the commonest UK strain).

Ref: Edwards & Bouchier. Davidsons Principles and Practice of Medicine. 17th edn. p 1094-5

ANSWER   64

A. TRUE   B. TRUE   C. TRUE   D. FALSE   E. FALSE

During sepsis and multiple organ failure there is loss of regulation of the immunoinflammatory cascade and activation or secretion of a massive range of mediators related to it:

i)   complement- activated both via the classical and alternate pathways.

ii) coagulation cascade- DIC, increases in factor XII, prekallikrien and bradykinin and activation of the intrinsic and extrinsic clotting system can all occur.

iii) platelets- release platelet activating factor, thromboxane A2, oxygen free radicals, serotonin and endoperoxides.

iv) cytokines- increased tumour necrosis factor and interleukins 1,6,8. Interleukin 10 may be regulatory acting as a modulator.

v)   lipid mediators- thromboxanes, prostacycline and the prostoglandins are released.

vi) proteases- elastase, collagenase and trypsin may increase. The antiprotease alpha 2 macroglobulin is reduced in these conditions.

vii) macophage-monocytes- activity increases producing oxygen free radicals, nitric oxide, cytokines and a variety of enzymes.

viii) polymorphonuclear leucocytes- produce oxygen free radicals, enzymes, inflammatory mediators including PAF and prostaglandins.

ix) endothelial cells- produce inflammatory mediators and adhesion molecules. They become procoagulant and lose their ability to produce thrombomodulin.

x)   lymphocytes- tend to be suppressed.

Ref: Deby-Dupont G, Lamy M. Mediators in critical illness. Current Anaesthesia and Critical Care 1995;6:3-9.

ANSWER   65

A. FALSE   B. FALSE   C. TRUE   D. TRUE   E. FALSE

Hypothermia is variably defined as a core temperature below 35-36°C. Amongst its effects at 30°C are unconciousness, a 50% reduction in cardiac output, and the presence of J waves in the ECG which are clinically insignificant. Apnoea does not occur until 24°C. Brown fat in infants contains numerous specialised mitochondria where uncoupled phosphorylation can occur and which can increase chemical thermogenesis by 100%. It is stimulated by the sympathetic nervous system in hypothermia.

Ref: Guyton & Hall. Textbook of Medical Physiology. Body temp, temperature reduction & fever.
Ref: Yentis, Hirsch, Smith. Anaesthesia A to Z. Hypothermia. Temperature regulation.

ANSWER   66

A. FALSE   B. TRUE   C. FALSE   D. TRUE   E. FALSE

There is no single tool for monitoring depth of anaesthesia and therefore for predicting likelihood of awareness. Guedel described his 4 stages with 4 planes to the third & surgical, stage of anaesthesia with subjects spontaneously breathing ether. Oesophageal contractions are increased by stress and decreased by anaesthesia. The frequency of ability to respond with movement to commands using the isolated forearm technique is variable, depending on anaesthetic technique, but has a poor correlation with ability to recall intra-operative events.

Cerebral function monitors representing a measure of the EEG are also crude in their attempts to demonstrate depth of anaesthesia.

Ref: Craft and Upton. Key topics in anaesthesia. Awareness and depth of anaesthesia.
Ref: Miller. Monitoring depth of anaesthesia.

ANSWER   67

A. FALSE   B. FALSE   C. TRUE   D. TRUE   E. FALSE

At the start of single lung ventilation the inspired FiO_2 should be increased to 50%. If arterial oxygen saturation cannot be maintained above 92% then further increases in FiO_2 should be tried, but awareness may become a problem if nitrous oxide is being used as part of the anaesthetic technique. If this still fails to raise the saturation then insufflation of oxygen to the collapsed lung, followed by the addition of CPAP and then PEEP to the ventilated lung should be tried. If all else fails, the collapsed lung may require re-inflation.

Ref. Miller RD. Anesthesia 3rd ed. Churchill Livingstone. Ch 50.

ANSWER   68

A. TRUE   B. FALSE   C. TRUE   D. FALSE   E. FALSE

In a Mapleson A system using controlled ventilation an expiratory pause is required to prevent rebreathing. Using a T piece the volume of the expiratory limb only needs to be the same as the tidal volume. In the heidbrink valve, the valve disc should be as light as possible to reduce resistance although this may increase sticking.

Ref. Ward. Balliere Tindall. Anaesthetic equipment. Chapter 7. Breathing attachments and their components.

ANSWER   69

A. FALSE   B. FALSE   C. TRUE   D. TRUE   E. TRUE

There are 3 common approaches to blocking the brachial plexus. The interscalene approach is ideal for shoulder and upper arm operations. It however frequently spares the C8 and T1 fibres which innervate the ulnar border of the forearm. Injection of local anaesthetic by this approach may produce cervical plexus block which may cause diaphragmatic paralysis. The phrenic nerve may also be blocked because of diffusion or inappropriate injection to the anterior side of the anterior scalene. The supraclavicular approach attempts to block the plexus at the first rib and is most reliable at producing anaesthesia of all four terminal nerves of the forearm and hand. It does however carry the greatest risk of pneumothorax. The axillary approach is simplest and has the least chance of pneumothorax. If paraesthesia cannot be elicited during this approach then one alternative is to delibarately pucture the axillary artery and advance the needle through the opposite wall where half the anaesthetic solution is deposited. The remainder is injected once the needle has been pulled back through the "anterior" wall of the artery.

Ref. Barash, Cullen and Stoelting. Clinical Anaesthesia. 2nd edition.J.B. Lippincott Company.

ANSWER   70

A. FALSE   B. TRUE   C. FALSE   D. TRUE   E. FALSE

The usual recording speed of an ECG is 25mm/s with a calibration of 1mV/cm. The PR interval is normally 0.12s-0.2s which represents 3 to 5 mm squares (each square represents 0.04s).

The normal axis lies between –30 degrees and +90 degrees. This is the summation of electrical potentials from the standard (I II III) and aVL leads plotted as vectors. The T wave is usually less than 5 mm in height. The unipolar chest leads VI to V6 are placed across the chest, V6 lies in the 5th intercostal space, midaxillary line.

Ref: Yentis, Hirsch, Smith. Anaesthesia A to Z. Butterworth Heinemann.

ANSWER 71

A. FALSE   B. FALSE   C. TRUE   D. TRUE   E. FALSE

In the foetus, oxygenated blood from the placenta passes through the single umbilical vein into the inferior vena cava. The right atrium is divided by the crista dividends which directs this blood into the left atrium via the foramen ovale. Hence it bypasses the right ventricle and the pulmonary vascular bed .It then progresses from the left atrium to the left ventricle and out through the ascending aorta to oxygenate the brain and upper extremities. Blood returns from the upper body to the right atrium via the superior vena cava where the crista dividends directs it into the right ventricle and hence into the pulmonary artery. Because of the resistance of the pulmonary vessels it passes from the pulmonary trunk to the aorta through the ductus arteriosus. This blood returns to the placenta via two umbilical arteries arising from the internal iliac arteries.

Ref. Barash, Cullen and Stoelting. Clinical Anaesthesia. 2nd edition. J.B. Lippincott Company.

ANSWER 72

A. FALSE   B. TRUE   C. FALSE   D. TRUE   E. TRUE

Following vascular injury, a platelet plug is formed. During this process ATP, ADP and 5HT are released from platelets. Collagen exposure and foreign materials result in the activation of the intrinsic pathway, which involves factors XII, XI, IX, VIII and calcium. The extrinsic pathway is activated by tissue thromboplastin. Normal haemostasis is a balance between coagulation and fibrinolysis.

Ref: Harrison , Healy and Thornton. AIDS to Anaesthesia. Churchill Livingstone.pp 196

ANSWER 73

A. TRUE   B. TRUE   C. TRUE   D. TRUE   E. TRUE

The lumbar plexus is formed by anterior divisions of L1 to L4. It is situated in the posterior part of the psoas muscle in front of the transverse processes of the lumbar vertebrae. The obturator nerve is a branch arising from L2, L3 and L4. It supplies the adductors of the thigh and the hip and knee joints. The iliohypogastric nerve arises from the first lumbar nerve. It communicates with the ilioinguinal nerve. The femoral nerve lies lateral to the artery and vein in the femoral sheath. It pierces the anterior part of the sheath and passes through fascia lata to supply skin on the anterior aspect of the thigh to midway between the pelvis and the knee. The ilioinguinal nerve supplies the upper, inner part of the thigh, the scrotum and the labia majora in the female.

Ref. Pick and Howden. Gray's Anatomy. Galley Press.

ANSWER 74

A. FALSE   B. TRUE   C. FALSE   D. FALSE   E. FALSE

The incidence of complications from central venous catheterisation is significantly higher if the cannula is in the right atrium and it should be correctly placed in the vena cava. The femoral route is often preferred due to the lower incidence of bleeding abnormalities (e.g. thrombocytopaenia). However it is associated with a greater degree of catheter colonisation, though the actual incidence of catheter-related sepsis is not increased. The a wave (due to atrial contraction) is not seen in atrial fibrillation. Giant a waves are seen when the right atrium contracts against a closed tricuspid valve in atrioventricular dissociation.

Ref: Clark, V.L. and Kruse, J.A. (1993) Vascular Procedures. In: Carlson, R.W. and Geheb, M.A. (Eds.) Principles and Practice of Medical Intensive Care, pp. 177-191. Philadelphia: W B Saunders

ANSWER 75

A. FALSE   B. FALSE   C. FALSE   D. TRUE   E. TRUE

Warfarin affects the post-ribosomal carboxylation of the glutamic acid residues of the precursors of clotting factors VII, IX, and X. The target range of the INR should be 3.0-4.5 for first generation mechanical valves (Starr-Edwards & Bjork-Shiley).For second generation mechanical valves the target INR should be 3.0-3.5 after mitral valve replacement and 2.5-3.0 after aortic valve replacement. The INR should be in the normal range for major surgery but should be adjusted to between 2.0-2.5 before planned dental procedures in order to reduce bleeding. In most cases, resumption of oral anticoagulant treatment is possible on the same day as the procedure and no interim heparin is necessary. Cardioversion of patients with atrial fibrillation who are not on anticoagulants is associated with systemic embolization in up to 7% therefore it is recommended that all patients with atrial fibrillation, even when it is of short duration, should be anticoagulated prior to cardioversion.

Ref: European Heart Journal 1995; 16, 1320-1330. Study Group of the Working Group on Valvular Heart Disease of the European Society of Cardiology. Guidelines for prevention of thromboembolic events in valvular heart disease.

ANSWER 76

A. TRUE   B. FALSE   C. FALSE   D. TRUE   E. TRUE

Patients with CRF are more sensitive to thiopentone, therefore a reduced rate of administration is the necessary step. Ketamine is possibly contraindicated due to its cardiovascular effects and the high incidence of CVS disease. Neuromuscular block onset times are not affected by CRF. The active metabolites are morphine-6-glucuronide and norpethidine.

Ref: Belani KG. Kidney transplantation. Int Anes Clinics 29.pp 17-39

ANSWER 77

A. TRUE   B. FALSE   C. TRUE   D. TRUE   E. TRUE

Every blood donation is tested for Hepatitis B surface Ag, Hepatits C viral Ab, and HIV 1 & 2 Ab's. Fresh Frozen Plasma carries the same risk as blood, and fibrinogen caries a 'high' risk since it is prepared from pooled plasma. The UK estimated risk for HIV transmission is less than 1/1,000,000 of blood component units transfused. Although the recently identified Hepatitis G virus has no donor screening test available it is likely that it is inactivated by plasma fractionation.

Ref: Yentis SM. Anaesthesia A to Z. Blood transfusion.
Ref: Handbook of transfusion medicine. HMSO.

ANSWER 78

A. FALSE   B. TRUE   C. FALSE   D. FALSE   E. FALSE

Despite the large number of modes of mechanical ventilation, there is often little evidence to prove the advantage of one over another. Most recommendations are therefore a combination of this evidence, theoretical advantages and clinical experience. IMV provides mandatory breaths interpersed with a facility for spontaneous ventilation. Therefore, this mode can be used for all patients from those fully ventilated to those breathing entirely spontaneously depending on the breath rate set. The disadvantages are that the work of breathing spontaneously may be high due to the resistance of the circuit, and a spontaneous inspiration immediately followed by a mandatory breath may cause 'breath stacking' and increase the chance of ventilator induced lung injury. This latter disadvantage is overcome with synchronised IMV- if the patient takes a spontaneous breath within a predetermined time from the next mandatory breath the mandatory breath is given as the patient inspires rather than following it. Mandatory minute volume ensures a predetermined minute volume whether spontaneous or mechanical. A major disadvantage is that a high respiratory rate/low tidal volume (and therefore inadequate alveolar ventilation) spontaneous ventilatory pattern may satisfy the minute volume specified. Pressure support ventilation (inspiratory assist, assisted spontaneous breathing) relies on the patient triggering the ventilator (by pressure, flow or rarely volume). A positive pressure breath is then given to a set inspiratory pressure and inspiration stops when the flow falls below a predetermined level. There is no strong evidence to support the use of a sigh breath which increases the tidal volume by 1.5 or 2 times.

Ref: Hillman and Bishop. Clinical Intensive Care. Cambridge University Press. Ch 20

ANSWER 79

A. TRUE   B. TRUE   C. TRUE   D. TRUE   E. TRUE

Nocturia is a symptom which may go unnoticed unless the patient is specifically questioned. The normocytic normochromic anaemia of renal failure is due to reduced erythropoietin production by the kidney. High urea levels (> 30 mmol / l) cause bone marrow toxicity and reduce red cell life. It is hence unresponsive to iron supplementation. Uraemia causes the skin to accumulate a yellow brown pigment and it becomes dry and itchy. Causes of pericarditis include viral infection, ischaemia, rheumatoid arthritis, TB, uraemia and SLE. Peripheral neuropathy is due to the accumulation of toxic metabolites associated with uraemia and so maybe reversed by dialysis.

Ref: Kumar & Clark. Clinical Medicine. Balliere Tindall. Chapter 9

ANSWER 80

A. TRUE   B. TRUE   C. TRUE   D. TRUE   E. TRUE

The surgical approach for oesophagectomy depends upon the site of the lesion. High tumours require a high midline laparotomy incision to mobilise the stomach followed by a right cervical incision and mobilisation of the upper oesophagous with subsequent pull-through. Middle tumours require a midline laparotomy followed by a right thoracotomy whereas low tumours require a left thoracoabdominal approach. It is useful to know the patients ultimate position on the table when considering lines etc. If a colonic interposition is planned the patient will have undergone bowel preparation.

Ref: Porton. Aids to Operative Surgery. Churchill Livingstone.

ANSWER   81

A. FALSE   B. FALSE   C. FALSE   D. TRUE   E. TRUE

Anxiety or agitation is experienced by an estimated 70-87% of patients in the ICU. The reasons are the underlying illness, therapeutic interventions and an altered sensorium. Limiting this stress response may improve a patient's ability to recover by reducing catecholamine and cortisol secretion, and allowing cooperation with procedures may reduce their inherent risks.

Non-pharmalogical methods to reduce anxiety must be carried out. These include interpersonal communication, environment improvement and optimal therapeutic regimens.

When drugs are used, pain must be considered first, and opioids are the commonest group to be used. However, they do have many side effects and their ability to delay enteral feeding should not be ignored. Regional anaesthesia and NSAIDs are possible, but contraindications to both often exist. Alpha 2 adrenergic agonists provide sedation, anxiolysis, hypnosis, analgesia and sympatholysis. However, they are limited by hypotension and bradycardia. Antihistamines can be used to depress CNS activity but are let down by their inconsistency, lack of controllability and antimuscarinic side effects. Barbiturates tend to be avoided as they accumulate but they are useful as anticonvulsants and in the management of raised intracranial pressure. Benzodiazepines bind to the GABA/benzodiazepine complex on neurones, increasing its binding affinity for the inhibitory transmitter GABA and hyperpolarizing the cell as intracellular chloride levels rise. Droperidol is a more potent alpha 1 adrenergic antagonist than haloperidol and therefore, when used for sedation, causes more hypotension. Both drugs can cause extrapyramidal symptoms and the neurolept malignant syndrome. Propofol supports the growth of bacteria and there are reports of bacteraemia due to contaminated infusions. Chloral hydrate, ketamine and volatile anaesthetic agents are also possible sedative agents that may be used.

Ref: Kovarik WD, Goldstein B. Pharmacological approach to sedation of the critically ill patient. Clinical Intensive Care 1996;7:248-257

ANSWER   82

A. FALSE   B. FALSE   C. FALSE   D. TRUE   E. FALSE

Magnetic resonance imaging involves placement of the patient within a powerful magnetic field causing alignment of atoms with an odd number of protons or neutrons. Radiofrequency pulses are then applied causing deflection of the atoms with absorption of energy. When these stop, the atoms return to their aligned position emitting energy as radiofrequency waves. These can be analysed to provide information about the make up of tissues. No X-rays are used.

The powerful magnets are not thought to cause direct harm. They may be switched off quickly in an emergency but require lengthy and expensive manoeuvres to be reset. The radiofrequency pulses may cause heating effects but this is insignificant.

Ref: Yentis, Hirsch, Smith. Anaesthesia A to z. Butterworth Heinemann.

ANSWER   83

A. TRUE   B. FALSE   C. TRUE   D. TRUE   E. TRUE

The highest temperature is normally recorded in the rectum and is 0.5 derees centigrade higher than the oesophageal. Both are taken as core temperatures. Resistance wire thermometers use platinum, copper or nickel whose resistance increases with increasing temperature and hence can be used to measure temperature electrically. Thermistor thermometers consist of semi-conductor fused heavy metal oxides such as cobalt, manganese and nickel whose resistance decreases with increasing temperature. They are composed of tiny beads making them ideal for temperature measurement in pulmonary artery catheters. Response times for electrical temperature probes depend on size, the smaller probe has a smaller heat capacity and therefore a shorter response time.

Ref: Principles of Measurement and Monitoring in Anaesthesia and Intensive Care. 3rd Edition. Sykes, Vickers, Hull. Blackwell Scientific Publications.

ANSWER 84

A. TRUE   B. FALSE   C. FALSE   D. TRUE   E. TRUE

Breast, lung, colo-rectal, pancreatic, stomach, testicular, uterine and ovarian tumours all commonly metastasise to liver. Prostate tumours commonly metastasise to bone and thyroid tumours metastasise to bone and lung.

Ref: McLatchie. Oxford Handbook of Clinical Surgery. Oxford University Press.

ANSWER 85

A. FALSE   B. TRUE   C. TRUE   D. TRUE   E. FALSE

Cerebral monitoring is aimed at assessing cerebral perfusion, metabolism or function. Xenon clearance was the first modality developed for clinical measurement of cerebral blood flow. TCD is of value to assess blood velocity in the Middle Cerebral Artery. It is used extensively to assess perfusion during carotid cross-clamping in carotid arterial reperfusion surgery. ICP monitoring is most valuable in head injuries where it is the gold standard for assessing the need for intervention. An ICP of >20 mmHg is normally used as a threshold for treatment. Jugular bulb oxygenation is an easy method for measuring global supply/demand balance, however it is not able to assess regional problems, particularly as there is a weighting toward the better per-fused tissues. EEG monitoring is used to assess cerebral function and will detect the secondary effects of a 50% reduction in cerebral perfusion.

Ref: Prough, D.S. (1993) Neurologic Monitoring. In: Carlson, R.W. and Geheb, M.A. (Eds.) Principles and Practice of Medical Intensive Care, pp. 221-234. Philadelphia: W B Saunders

ANSWER 86

A. TRUE   B. TRUE   C. TRUE   D. TRUE   E. TRUE

The internal jugular vein is a continuation of the sigmoid sinus and begins at the jugular foramen. Its tributaries include the inferior petrosal sinus, facial, pharyngeal, lingual, superior thyroid , middle thyroid, and occipital veins. In the neck it travels lateral to the internal carotid artery in the carotid sheath. It drains the scalp and face .

Ref: Snell. Clinical Anatomy For Medical Students. Little Brown. Boston.

ANSWER 87

A. TRUE   B. FALSE   C. FALSE   D. FALSE   E. TRUE

The treatment of ARDS remains controversial due to a lack of evidence. This partly relates to the poorly standardised definition which also makes it difficult to see if mortality rates are reducing. Theoretically, overenthusiastic fluid administration will exacerbate pulmonary oedema. There is now evidence to suggest that this occurs in practice. Inhaled nitric oxide at concentrations of up to 40 ppm (and most commonly 2-12 ppm) improves V/Q matching by selectively dilating blood vessels being ventilated. It also tends to reduce pulmonary artery pressure and improve right ventricular function, although does not return the former to normal values. There is no evidence to show it reduces mortality despite the often dramatic improvements in oxygenation. Several reports show the benefit in oxygenation of the prone position in ARDS although again effect on outcome is unknown. The improvement can be dramatic although not all patients respond and the manoeuvre may not be wise in very unstable patients (who conversely may be those most likely to benefit). During the late fibroproliferative phase of ARDS, PEEP requirements usually decrease but a certain level often has to be maintained. There are some descriptive studies indicating that corticosteroids in this phase may be beneficial.

Ref: Bone RC, Vincent JL (Eds). Current Opinion in Critical Care. 1996;2.

ANSWER 88

A. FALSE   B. FALSE   C. TRUE   D. TRUE   E. TRUE

The first three letters defining pacemakers apply to the chamber paced, chamber sensed and the response. The fourth and fifth letters apply to programability and anti-arrythmic features of the pacemaker. Pacemaker function and threshold for capture can be affected by the volatile agents. Pacemakers which have been reset to basal VOO mode are more prone to being adversely affected in relation to their programming by external stimuli. Rate responsive pacemakers can increase their paced rate in response to rises in contractility as might be produced by increased sympathetic tone.

Ref: Craft & Upton. Key topics in Anaesthesia. Pacemakers.
Ref: Miller. Anesthesia. Pacemakers.

ANSWER 89

A. TRUE   B. FALSE   C. TRUE   D. TRUE   E. FALSE

Omeprazole is a proton pump inhibitor and like the H_2-receptor antagonists it reduces some hepatic drug metabolism by inhibition of the cytochrome P450 system. Cimetidine and omeprazole have the highest affinity, while ranitidine has only 1/6 the effect. The following are recognised interactions:-

Phenytoin	- effects enhanced by omeprazole
Warfarin	- effects enhanced by omeprazole
Diazepam	- effects enhanced by omeprazole
Ketoconazole	- absorption reduced by omeprazole
Aminophylline	- effects enhanced by omeprazole

Sucralfate, used for gut mucosal protection particularly in intensive care units, contains aluminium which results in intra-luminal binding and formation of ion complexes with ciprofloxacin, tetracycline, digoxin, quinidine, thyroxine, ketoconazole, phenytoin and possibly warfarin.

Ref: Current Anaesthesia and Critical Care. Churchill Livingstone. 1995. Vol 6, No 2, 103-112. Drug interactions and anaesthesia. BNF. Pharmaceutical Press. 1996, No 31, Appendix 1.

ANSWER 90

A. TRUE   B. TRUE   C. FALSE   D. FALSE   E. FALSE

A pulmonary capillary wedge pressure (PCWP) greater than the pulmonary artery end diastolic pressure (PAEDP) suggests that the pulmonary artery catheter tip is not in West zone III. This is the zone where the pulmonary artery and venous pressures exceed the alveolar pressures allowing for uninterrupted blood flow and a continuous communication with distal intracardiac pressures. Usually the catheter, being flow directed, is directed to this zone since this is where there is greatest flow. PEEP alters ventricular distensibility and reduces venous return which causes a disproportionate increase in PCWP (and LVEDP). Ventilator disconnection is not recommended during PEEP as this results in haemodynamic changes and hypoxaemia. Left atrial pressure is assumed to reflect LVEDP. Obstruction at the mitral valve (stenosis, myxoma or clot) can interfere with this relationship. Tachycardia shortens ventricular diastole reducing distal runoff of pulmonary blood flow and thereby increasing pulmonary vascular resistances. Hence the PAEDP cannot be assumed to reflect distal diastolic pressures including the PCWP.

Ref: Barash, Cullen, Stoelting. Clinical Anesthesia. 2nd Edition. J.B. Lippincott Company.

QUESTION 1

The following intravenous solutions have a pH greater than 6

A. 5% Dextrose
B. Ringer's Lactate
C. 0.9% Saline
D. Haemaccel
E. Hespan

QUESTION 2

Concerning the management of tachyarrhythmias

A. Medical cardioversion of acute atrial fibrillation can be done using a flecainide infusion 10 mg/kg
B. Rapid atrial pacing for 30 – 60 seconds frequently restores sinus rhythm in atrial flutter
C. 80% of patients with Woolf-Parkinson-White syndrome experience arrhythmias
D. Treatment of torsades de pointes may involve pacing or an isoprenaline infusion
E. Treatment of torsades de pointes consists of prolonging the QT interval

QUESTION 3

In an infant with tetralogy of fallot undergoing cardiac catheterisation

A. A decreased pulmonary blood flow is usually present
B. Augmenting right ventricular contractility is important to maintain cardiac output
C. A decreased systemic vascular resistance is important to reduce left ventricular oxygen demand
D. Nitric oxide is now a mainstay in augmenting right ventricular emptying
E. If hypovolaemia occurs, fluid boluses should be given as blood to maintain a high PCV

QUESTION 4

Concerning immunodeficiency diseases

A. Most immunodeficiency syndromes are due to a single defect
B. Isolated IgA deficiency is often asymptomatic
C. A thymoma must be suspected when a patient over 40 years develops hypogammaglobulinaemia
D. Systemic lupus erythematosus may cause septicaemia due to excessive complement consumption
E. Primary hypogammaglobulinaemia results in recurrent infections with protozoa and mycobacteria

QUESTION 5

In a patient having a transurethral resection of prostate

A. Ethanol added to the irrigant can be measured in the drainage fluid to estimate fluid absorption
B. Saline disturbs the use of current with the resectoscope
C. Absorption is reduced to a safer level by not placing the irrigant more than 1.5m above the patient
D. Mannitol and sorbitol can be used to make the irigation fluid isotonic
E. Glycine is a stimulatory neurotransmitter putting patients at risk of convulsions

QUESTION 6

The use of scavenging of anaesthetic gases includes

A. Passive systems with a reservoir bag to accomodate high expiratory flow rates
B. Semi active systems employing a venturi system
C. Aldasorbers to absorb halothane using activated charcoal
D. A collecting system with a 22mm fitting from the expiratory port of the breathing system
E. A maximum of 25ppm for theatre concentration of halogenated vapours

QUESTION 7

Pulmonary artery flow-directed catheters (Swan-Ganz catheters)

A. Have been shown to be detrimental to many patients in high dependency care
B. Measure left atrial pressure directly
C. Allow accurate measurement of cardiac output in patients with tricuspid regurgitation
D. Will underestimate cardiac output if less than the required volume of saline is used
E. In spontaneously breathing patients pressures should be measured in inspiration

QUESTION 8

The following agents decrease cerebral blood flow (CBF) and cerebral metabolic rate for oxygen (CMRO$_2$)

- **A.** Dopamine
- **B.** Sufentanil
- **C.** Althesin
- **D.** Isoflurane
- **E.** Diazepam

QUESTION 9

Concerning severity of illness scoring systems

- **A.** TISS assumes that illness severity is directly related to treatment and monitoring
- **B.** The Simplified Acute Physiology Score (SAPS II) does not incorporate age
- **C.** APACHE II has a weighting applied to the relative abnormality of each physiological variable
- **D.** The trauma score measures more variables than the revised trauma score
- **E.** APACHE II is calculated from the best physiological values

QUESTION 10

Haemodialysis enhances the elimination of the following drugs taken in overdose

- **A.** Theophylline
- **B.** Phenobarbitone
- **C.** Aspirin
- **D.** Ethylene glycol
- **E.** Lithium

QUESTION 11

An adult patient with trisomy 21 is scheduled for a tonsillectomy

- **A.** The presence of a small mouth often makes laryngoscopy difficult
- **B.** There is an increased incidence of sub-glottic stenosis
- **C.** Atlanto-axial instability, if present, is usually asymptomatic
- **D.** An endocardial cushion defect is the most likely cardiac abnormality
- **E.** An increased sensitivity to opiates is to be expected

QUESTION 12

Concerning hypovolaemic shock

A. Colloids decrease mortality relative to crystalloids when used as the resuscitating fluid
B. If it occurs in trauma victims then the mortality is doubled
C. Bicarbonate should be given to correct acidosis
D. Mannitol improves renal perfusion and can prevent the development of acute renal failure (ARF)
E. Glomerular filtration rate (GFR) falls early

QUESTION 13

The following drugs may increase body temperature

A. Clindamycin
B. Streptokinase
C. Bleomycin
D. Atropine
E. Hydralazine

QUESTION 14

Concerning direct pressure monitoring

A. Systolic pressure is more accurately recorded than mean pressure
B. Bubbles in the tubing tend to produce an underdamped trace
C. Bubbles in the tubing tend to reduce the natural frequency of the system
D. Kinking of the tubing will reduce the natural frequency of the system
E. A system with a high natural frequency gives more accurate reproduction of pressures associated with a rapid heart rate

QUESTION 15

Concerning liver transplantation

A. Isolated unresectable liver tumour is not an indication
B. Venevenous bypass is usually employed in adults
C. Calcium infusion is required during the anhepatic phase
D. Hypokalaemia occurs at the time of reperfusion
E. Nitrous oxide should be avoided

QUESTION 16

The non articular manifestations of rheumatoid arthritis include

A. Cardiac tamponade
B. Sarcoidosis of the kidney
C. Caplans syndrome
D. Ankle oedema
E. A glove and stocking sensory loss

QUESTION 17

When assessing a patient with burns

A. First degree burns are characterised by blisters
B. The head of an adult represents approximately 18% of the body surface
C. Carbon deposits in the pharynx suggest inhalational burn
D. Rhabdomyolysis does not occur with electrical burns
E. In children a urine output of 1ml/kg/hr is the aim when infusing fluid

QUESTION 18

In a patient with sickle cell disease

A. There is correspondingly more protection against falciparum malaria than in those with sickle cell trait
B. Anaemia is present from birth
C. Cardiomegaly is a feature
D. Sickling crises are precipitated by the cold
E. Life expectancy is reduced in the UK

QUESTION 19

Inhaled anaesthetic agents

A. Play a part in the increased venous admixture seen in ventilated patients
B. Are responsible for the raised $PaCO_2$ seen in spontaneously breathing patients
C. Cause an increase in airways resistance
D. Improve total lung compliance
E. Have no effect on the muscles of respiration

QUESTION 20

Carcinoma of the oesophagus

A. Is usually adenocarcinoma
B. Is associated with Plummer Vinson syndrome
C. Causes tracheo-oesophageal fistula
D. Primary spread is blood-borne
E. Hoarseness is a feature

QUESTION 21

Diverticular disease

A. Usually affects the rectum
B. Is common in patients < 35 years old
C. Classically causes right iliac fossa pain
D. Is unusual if the patient eats a high-fibre diet
E. Presents with per-rectal bleeding

QUESTION 22

Concerning the cardiac action potential

A. In the sino-atrial node automaticity is partly determined by inward Ca^{++} flux
B. Inward Ca^{++} flux occurs throughout phases 1,2 and 3
C. Conduction is fastest through the atrio-ventricular node
D. Isoflurane slows phase 4 repolarisation in an isolated heart
E. Resting membrane potential is mainly determined by potassium

QUESTION 23

The Post Tetanic Count

A. Should be preceded by a single 50Hz stimulus
B. Should be preceded by a tetanic stimulus of 3 seconds duration
C. Counts twitches in response to stimuli delivered at 1 second intervals
D. Should commence after a 3 second pause following tetanic stimulation
E. Is directly related to the intensity of the block

QUESTION 24

In a patient with severe rheumatoid disease having a total hip replacement

A. Sensory evoked potentials may add to the safety of the procedure
B. Vertebral fracture and cord injury may result from a regional anaesthetic procedure
C. Crico-arytenoid disease is rare
D. Respiratory compliance will be limited mainly by lung fibrosis
E. Cardiovascular disease is usually vasculitic in origin

QUESTION 25

In patients who present for renal transplantation

A. Spousal related donor grafts have worse one year prognoses than living related donor grafts
B. Only size match and blood group compatibility are required for cadaveric grafts
C. Cyclosporin is the most common cause of post transplantation convulsions
D. Patients are at high risk of bony injuries during positioning
E. Epidural is the analgesic technique of choice

QUESTION 26

In the management of a patient with a thermal injury

A. Suxamethonium does not produce a hyperkalaemic response within the 24 hours after a major burn
B. Suxamethonium is principally dangerous due to the proliferation in junctional acetylcholine receptors
C. Decreased sensitivity to non-depolarising relaxants is seen
D. An increased metabolism of narcotics is seen
E. Bronchial and bronchiolar damage is largely caused by agents within inhaled smoke rather than by a direct thermal effect

QUESTION 27

Complications post-oesophagectomy include

A. Pleural effusion
B. Atrial fibrillation in 10 -20% patients
C. Delayed gastric emptying
D. Pneumothorax
E. Mediastinitis

QUESTION 28

The following associations are correct

A. Infra-red absorption used in capnography
B. Fuel cell used in oxygen measurements
C. Delta waves in EEG present during sleep
D. Train of four stimulation is four pulses at 50 Hz
E. Surface tension measured in N/m

QUESTION 29

In a patient who fails to show sufficient neuromuscular function at the end of anaesthesia

A. If aminoglycosides are implicated then calcium therapy may improve NM function
B. Double burst stimulation at an interval of 750 msecs may demonstrate fade
C. Dual block may be due to mixed use of depolarising and non depolarising agents
D. Post tetanic count of <5 indicates adequate reversal
E. Head lift for 5 seconds implies that >30% neuromuscular block is present

QUESTION 30

Acute liver failure

A. Due to viral hepatitis is most commonly due to hepatitis B
B. Is complicated by sepsis in up to 80% of patients
C. Due to paracetamol is more likely in alcoholics
D. Has a higher mortality if associated with low factor V levels
E. Should be monitored by serial aspartate transaminase (AST) levels to assess the course of the disease

QUESTION 31

The following infection/antibiotic combinations are appropriate

A. Multi resistant Staphylococcus aureus and vancomycin
B. Streptococcus pneumoniae and penicillin
C. Enterococci and gentamicin
D. Multi resistant Staphylococcus aureus and gentamicin
E. Acenetobacter spp and imipenem

QUESTION 32

Epidural Analgesia

A. Epidural opioids have a lower incidence of side-effects than other routes in the control of pain in terminal care

B. Pruritis is seen in patients treated with local anaesthetic alone

C. Epidural morphine is associated with respiratory depression especially 6 to 12 hours after administration

D. The efficacy of local anaesthetics and opioids are enhanced by the addition of clonidine

E. Placental transfer of opioid is prevented by use of epidural rather than intramuscular opioids

QUESTION 33

A patient's cervical spine can be 'cleared' by the ITU resident following normal

A. A-P radiograph of the C-spine down to C7-T1

B. CT of neck

C. Examination of the sedated patient

D. Peripheral nerve stimulation

E. Three view radiographs (A-P, lateral, open mouth)

QUESTION 34

Arterial blood gas analysis

A. The presence of air bubbles may cause either an increase or a decrease in PO_2

B. Placing the syringe in a bag containing ice cubes ensures that the sample is rapidly cooled to 0 degrees Centigrade

C. Excessive heparin in the sample will cause a fall in the bicarbonate value from the machine

D. Sodium heparin has a pH of 5.0 - 7.0

E. Halothane may lead to an inaccurately high PO_2

QUESTION 35

Concerning nutritional support for patients with chronic obstructive pulmonary disease (COPD)

A. Impaired nutrition can result in reduced surfactant production

B. A high carbohydrate diet is preferred

C. Excessive protein intake worsens ventilatory drive

D. Pulmocare contains more than twice the fat content of Ensure

E. Pulmocare improves outcome compared to Ensure or Osmolite

QUESTION 36

In acute diabetic ketoacidosis

A. 0.9% saline should only be given once central venous pressure has been measured
B. A total body deficit of potassium is present
C. Gastric dilatation is a feature
D. Coma maybe the presenting feature
E. Hyperphosphataemia occurs

QUESTION 37

The brachial plexus

A. Roots lie deep to scalenus anterior
B. The supraclavicular approach allows total anaesthesia of the arm if successful
C. Gives origin to the musculocutaneous nerve of the arm
D. Block by the intrascalene approach will block the suprascapular nerves
E. Cords lie in the anterior triangle of the neck

QUESTION 38

The following are SI units

A. Ampere
B. Hour
C. Gramme
D. Kelvin
E. Candela

QUESTION 39

During the treatment of severe head trauma

A. Fluid restriction is essential to improve outcome
B. Routine prescription of corticosteroids is necessary
C. Hyperventilation to $PaCO_2$ levels less than 25 mmHg have been shown to worsen outcome
D. Immediate transfer to a neurosurgical unit should be arranged
E. Prophylactic antibodies should be given to those with basal skull fractures

QUESTION 40

The following are recognised causes of muscle weakness in the critically ill patient

A. Disuse atrophy
B. Hypomagnesaemia
C. Hypophosphataemia
D. Physiotherapy
E. Corticosteroid administration

QUESTION 41

In the resuscitation of a term neonate

A. The first step is to provide oxygen via a face mask
B. Adrenaline is indicated if if the heart rate is less than 80 beats/minute despite oxygenation
C. If given, the dose of adrenaline is 5 mcg / kg iv
D. Meconium is present in the amniotic fluid of 10-20% of newborns
E. A systolic blood pressure of 40 mmHg would be normal

QUESTION 42

In control of the systemic microcirculation

A. Neural input into the resistance vessels of different organs varies
B. Renal arterioles have low tone and therefore have little capacity to dilate
C. In the skin whilst resting tone is high there is a dilator and constrictor capacity
D. Inhibition of NO synthase produces equal increases in vascular resistance in different tissues
E. 70% of blood volume at rest is in the venous circulation with the majority in venules

QUESTION 43

During aortic aneurysm surgery

A. Invasive arterial pressure should be monitored at induction
B. The use of frusemide increases renal oxygen consumption
C. In thoracoabdominal repair slight hyperglycaemia is beneficial
D. Hypotension after cross–clamp release is due to inadequate intravascular volume
E. Postoperative ventilation is mandatory

QUESTION 44

Cerebral blood flow is

A. Decreased by morphine
B. Decreased by propofol
C. Increased by thiopentone
D. Is not altered by fentanyl
E. Increased more by isoflurane than by halothane

QUESTION 45

The hepatorenal syndrome is characterized by

A. Sodium loss
B. Increased production of thromboxane
C. Increased production of nitric oxide
D. Renal vasodilatation
E. Return of normal renal function following liver transplantation

QUESTION 46

Following surgery, the secretion of antidiuretic hormone

A. Decreases the volume of urine passed
B. Decreases the osmolarity of urine
C. Increases the total amount of electrolyte free water in the body
D. Increases the reabsorption of water in the proximal tubule
E. Is the cause of a negative nitrogen balance

QUESTION 47

Hepatobiliary complications of total parenteral nutrition (TPN)

A. Include gallstone formation
B. Causing liver enzyme elevations are relentless in their progression
C. Indicate the need for immediate cessation of TPN
D. Often differ in their type according to the age of the patient
E. Can involve cholestasis

QUESTION 48

The following occur more commonly post-gastrectomy

A. Vitamin B12 and folate deficiency
B. Hypercalcaemia
C. Iron deficiency
D. Constipation
E. Pancreatitis

QUESTION 49

Thallium-201

A. Is a calcium analogue
B. Is used to demonstrate regional wall motion abnormalities
C. Is taken up predominantly by red blood cells
D. Will demonstrate areas of poor myocardial perfusion
E. Is used in combination with dobutamine to demonstrate "steal"

QUESTION 50

Intracranial pressure (ICP)

A. Reduction by thiopentone is due to vasodilatation-induced hypothermia
B. Can be reduced more effectively with mannitol+frusemide than with mannitol alone
C. Is unaffected by the administration of nitrous oxide
D. Manipulation using mannitol relies on an intact blood brain barrier
E. Is significantly reduced following the administration of opioids

QUESTION 51

Considering maternal extradural analgesia

A. There is less placental transfer of local anaesthetic in the presence of foetal acidosis
B. It abolishes the hyperventilation associated with labour
C. It increases uterine blood flow
D. It reduces perinatal morbidity and mortality for breech presentations
E. Use of lignocaine is associated with worse neonatal neurobehaviour scores than bupivacaine

QUESTION 52

Considering ketone bodies

A. The majority of amino acids can be converted into acetoacetate
B. The liver converts fatty acids into acetoacetate for transport to other parts of the body
C. Ketosis can arise from a diet composed almost entirely of fat
D. Citrate availability limits entry of acetyl-CoA into the citric acid cycle
E. A ketoacidosis causes hyponatraemia

QUESTION 53

Measurement of exhaled gases

A. Raman scattering allows measurement of nitrogen
B. Infra-red absorption allows measurement of oxygen
C. Mass spectrometry allows differentiation of different volatile anaesthetic agents
D. Calorimetric assay of CO_2 allows extremely accurate measurement suitable for research purposes
E. When using mass spectrometry, the gas should not be returned to the breathing system

QUESTION 54

Heparin

  A. Is a naturally occurring anticoagulant

  B. Raises plasma triglyceride levels

  C. May cause Type II hypersensitivity reactions

  D. Is reversed by protamine due to drug displacement

  E. Inactivates thrombin by encouraging the action of antithrombin III

QUESTION 55

Auto-PEEP during mechanical ventilation

  A. Can be measured by subtracting set PEEP from the airway pressure measured during an inspiratory hold procedure

  B. Is suggested by a continued expiratory flow at end expiration on a flow-time monitor

  C. May reduce minute volume in volume control ventilation

  D. Is more likely to occur with inverse ratio compared to conventional ratio ventilation

  E. Increases in likelihood as the minute volume increases

QUESTION 56

Concerning the pharmacological control of blood sugar

  A. The sulphonylureas act by displacing bound insulin from the beta cells of the islets of Langerhans

  B. The chronic administration of tolbutamide is associated with alcohol intolerance

  C. Metformin lowers plasma cholesterol, triglycerides and low-density lipoproteins

  D. Chlorpropramide needs to be omitted only on the day of surgery

  E. Halothane worsens glycaemic control

QUESTION 57

Ulcerative colitis is associated with

  A. Cholangitis

  B. Pyoderma gangrenosum

  C. Moniliasis of the mouth

  D. Ankylosing spondylitis

  E. Clubbing

QUESTION 58

The potential advantages of pressure controlled ventilation over traditional volume controlled ventilation are

A. Mean airway pressure is reduced
B. Peak alveolar pressure is limited
C. More accurate control of minute volume
D. The shape of the inspiratory flow waveform can be altered
E. A reduction of the shearing forces that occur at the onset of inspiration

QUESTION 59

Acute bacterial meningitis

A. Impairs cerebral autoregulation
B. Due to Strep. pneumoniae can be treated with vancomycin and rifampicin
C. Must always be treated with corticosteroids in addition to antibiotics
D. May necessitate tracheal intubation due to seizures
E. Should always be confirmed by examination of cerebrospinal fluid

QUESTION 60

The following may mimic an acute abdomen

A. Diabetic ketoacidosis
B. Acute intermittent porphyria
C. Myocardial infarction
D. Sickle cell crisis
E. Phaeochromocytoma

QUESTION 61

Concerning the prevention af acute renal failure (ARF)

A. Dopamine in low doses acts mainly by increasing the glomerular filtration rate (GFR)
B. Mannitol helps prevent ARF in jaundiced patients undergoing surgery
C. Noradrenaline decreases the incidence of ARF in septic patients
D. Frusemide reduces oxygen consumption in the proximal renal tubules
E. The Charing Cross protocol = aggressive fluid therapy, PA catheter monitoring, noradrenaline, GTN and frusemide infusions

QUESTION 62

Capnographic monitoring

A. A raised baseline may be normal in a sidestream analyser monitoring an 8kg child

B. An increase in the respiratory dead space may cause a fall in the plateau phase

C. Oesophageal intubation is excluded by a pulsatile carbon dioxide trace

D. In respiratory disease the end-tidal carbon dioxide is an accurate indicator of $PaCO_2$

E. After sudden ventricular fibrillation end-tidal carbon dioxide falls gradually until successful resuscitation is commenced

QUESTION 63

In a patient with a breast lump

A. Skin tethering suggests carcinoma

B. Excision is mandatory

C. Oestrogen therapy is of use

D. If mobile and discreet, it may be just observed

E. Disappearance may occur after aspiration

QUESTION 64

The following clinical associations are correct

A. Plasma potassium 2.6 mmol/l - ST depression on ECG

B. Plasma sodium 114 mmol/l - bronchial carcinoma

C. Plasma calcium (corrected) 3 mmol/l - prolonged QT interval on ECG

D. CSF glucose 1 mmol/l with plasma glucose 6 mmol/l - bacterial meningitis

E. Serum albumin 60 g/l - trauma

QUESTION 65

In mitral stenosis

A. Haemoptysis is a feature

B. Rheumatic heart disease is always the cause

C. Pleural effusions may occur secondary to sodium retention

D. Prophylactic antibiotics for dental treatment are unnecessary in mild, asymptomatic cases

E. Anticoagulation can be part of management

QUESTION 66

Hypoglycaemia is found in

A. Hypopituitarism
B. Cirrhosis of the liver
C. Post gastrectomy
D. Hyperadrenalism
E. Insulinoma

QUESTION 67

Concerning brain–stem death and organ donation

A. Age 56 precludes cardiac donation
B. An isoelectric EEG should be present upon diagnosis of brain-stem death
C. Primary CNS malignancy precludes organ donation
D. Donor spinal reflexes are no longer present
E. Spontaneous ventilation may be present in the donor

QUESTION 68

The following combinations may give rise to drug interactions beyond summative effects

A. Tranylcypromine and selective serotonin reuptake inhibitors (SSRI's)
B. Carbamazepine and tricyclic antidepressants
C. Propofol and fentanyl
D. Lignocaine and opioid analgesics
E. Verapamil and benzodiazepines

QUESTION 69

In hepatocellular failure

A. Diuretic therapy may precipitate hepatic encephalopathy
B. Complicated by encephalopathy, lactulose administration is routine
C. Protein intake is routinely restricted
D. Folate administration should be continued indefinitely
E. Vitamin K administration readily reverses prothrombin time prolongation

QUESTION 70

Pyloric stenosis is characterised by

A. A preponderance of male sufferers
B. Metabolic alkalosis
C. Raised aldosterone secretion
D. Hyperkalaemia
E. An alkalotic urine

QUESTION 71

When treating cancer pain

A. Opioids should only be given when the pain re-emerges
B. The initial drug used for nociceptive pain should be a weak opioid such as codeine
C. Rectal morphine can be used at 2-3 times the injectable dose
D. Corticosteroids are only used if an intracerebral tumour causes pain secondary to raised intracranial pressure
E. Motor nerve damage secondary to phenol will last longer than that due to alcohol

QUESTION 72

The following are common problems in patients with end stage renal failure

A. Postural hypotension
B. Electrolyte imbalance and alkalosis
C. Relative thrombocytopenia
D. Ischaemic cardiomyopathy
E. Chronic sub acute bacterial peritonitis

QUESTION 73

In a clinical trial with two treatment arms, randomisation means

A. Treatments are chosen in relation to some predictable event
B. Results are treated in random order
C. Results are analysed usng the chi-squared test
D. Treatments are allocated by reference to a series of random numbers
E. Therapy is allocated by an independent person

QUESTION 74

The following are correct innervations

A. Lateral rectus : abducent nerve
B. Mucous membrane of the floor of the mouth : lingual nerve
C. Skin over palmar lateral three and a half digits : ulnar nerve
D. Pudenal nerve : glans of the penis
E. Auriculotemporal nerve : temporomandibular joint

QUESTION 75

Regarding the blood supply to the spinal cord

A. The anterior spinal artery supplies the anterior third
B. The posterior spinal artery arises from the vertebral artery
C. The artery of Adamkiewicz is more common on the right
D. There is one posterior spinal artey
E. The only direct supply comes from the anterior and posterior spinal arteries

QUESTION 76

To be able to confirm brain stem death in a patient

A. Two senior physicians must conduct the test together
B. During the cold caloric test the eyes move away from the side of the stimulus
C. The cause of irreversible coma must be known
D. The arterial $PaCO_2$ must rise to above 50 mmHg during the apnoea test
E. The patients EEG is isoelectric

QUESTION 77

For surgery confined to the foot

A. Spinal anaesthesia to the level of L4 will be adequate
B. The saphenous nerve supplies the medial side of the ankle joint
C. The deep peroneal nerve supplies the second and third toes
D. The tibial nerve supplies the sole of the foot
E. 6 nerves need to be blocked at the ankle

QUESTION 78

In atrial fibrillation (AF)

A. Thyrotoxicosis is a cause
B. Anticoagulation is only advised for those with chronic AF
C. The ECG shows ' f ' waves
D. Alcohol toxicity is a cause
E. Flecainide can be used to treat paroxysmal AF

QUESTION 79

Concerning the carotid arteries

A. The left common carotid artery arises from the brachiocephalic artery
B. The division of the common carotids into external and internal carotids occurs at the level of C6
C. The internal carotid gives rise to the the middle and anterior cerebral arteries
D. The carotid sinus is a dilatation of the internal carotid
E. The internal carotid gives rise to the vertebral artery

QUESTION 80

Considering the use of the laryngeal mask airway

A. The size two and a half mask is appropriate for patients of 20-30 Kg
B. The size one mask is not appropriate for children less than 4.5 Kg
C. The laryngeal mask cuff should be partly deflated prior to an autoclave cycle
D. The appropriate inflation volume for a size 2 mask is up to 25 mls
E. The appropriate inflation volume for a size 1 mask is less than 4 mls

QUESTION 81

Sodium reabsorption in the kidney is

A. Greater in the distal than in the proximal convoluted tubule
B. Only achieved in exchange for potassium excretion
C. The main objective of the countercurrent multiplier system
D. The major energy consuming activity of the kidney
E. Dependent upon on the glomerular filtration rate as well as aldosterone

QUESTION 82

Concerning the management of 'pre-eclampsia'

A. Low dose aspirin does not significantly reduce the incidence of pre-eclampsia
B. When methyldopa fails to control hypertension ACE inhibitors are indicated
C. The side effects of hydralazine may mimic the symptoms of impending eclampsia
D. In severe pre-eclampsia the wedge pressure (PCWP) is usually elevated
E. Magnesium sulphate toxicity can be treated with intra venous calcium gluconate

QUESTION 83

In the jugular venous pulse

A. The y descent precedes the v wave
B. The c wave corresponds to bulging of the tricuspid valve into the right atrium
C. The x wave occurs during systole
D. Cannon waves occur with atrial contraction on a closed tricuspid valve
E. The x wave is lost in tricuspid valve regurgitation

QUESTION 84

During the measurement of cardiac output

A. Indocyanine blue is commonly used
B. The thermal indicator dilution method is prone to recirculation error
C. There are normal fluctuations in pulmonary blood temperature between inspiration and expiration
D. Doppler ultrasonography is more accurate than thermodilution
E. The thermistor of a pulmonary artery catheter is situated in the pulmonary artery for the thermal dilution method

QUESTION 85

The diaphragm

A. Has a central muscular trefoil
B. Is attached to the sides of the first to third lumbar vertebra on the left
C. Transmits the aorta at a level of the tenth thoracic vertebra
D. Transmits the oesophagus and the thoracic duct at the same opening
E. Derives a sensory and motor nervous supply from the phrenic nerve

QUESTION 86

Pulmonary artery wedge pressure does not reflect LVEDV in the following circumstances

A. Poor ventricular wall compliance
B. Pulmonary artery catheter tip too far advanced
C. Tricuspid regurgitation
D. Positive end expiratory pressure (PEEP)
E. Positive pressure ventilation

QUESTION 87

Congenital pyloric stenosis

A. Affects ~20 children in 1000 live births
B. Has equal sex incidence
C. Usually presents within 48hrs of birth
D. Presents with a palpable tumour
E. Presents with poor feeding

QUESTION 88

Normochromic normocytic anaemia usually occurs in

A. Rheumatoid arthritis
B. SLE
C. Vegans
D. Alcoholism
E. Neoplasia

QUESTION 89

The following drugs have >50% oral bioavailability

A. Disopyramide
B. Propranolol
C. Verapamil
D. Digoxin
E. Amiodarone

QUESTION 90

Regarding blood

A. Erythrocyte production is confined to the bone marrow and spleen in adults
B. Erythropoietin levels are increased in patients in renal failure
C. Vitamin B12 is required for normal red cell function
D. The life span of a red blood cell is about 120 days
E. Hypoxia is a major stimulus for the production of erythrocytes

Exam 5: Answers

QUESTION 1

A. FALSE   B. TRUE   C. FALSE   D. TRUE   E. FALSE

The actual pH of these solutions are:-

5% Dextrose	4.0
Ringer's Lactate	6.5
0.9% Saline	5.0
Haemaccel	7.3
Hespan	5.5

Ref: Care of the Critically Ill 1995; Vol 11, No 3, pg 114-119. Crystalloids and colloids in the critically ill patient. ABPI Data Sheet Compendium 1996 pgs 510 & 672

QUESTION 2

A. FALSE   B. TRUE   C. FALSE   D. TRUE   E. FALSE

The dose of flecainide for medical cardioversion is 2mg/kg over 15-30 mins. 60% of WPW patients experience arrhythmias. Treatment of torsades de pointes consists of reversing the underlying cause if possible and raising the heart rate by either pacing or isoprenaline infusion.

Ref: Current Anaesthesia and Critical Care 1995; Vol6, No 3: pg 155-161. Diagnosis and management of tachyarrhythmias

QUESTION 3

A. TRUE   B. FALSE   C. FALSE   D. FALSE   E. FALSE

Fallots tetralogy is a VSD, overriding aorta, right ventricular outflow obstruction and right ventricular hypertrophy. Pulmonary blood flow is usually decreased due to right ventricular outflow tract obstruction and any increase in right ventricular contractility usually worsens this due to dynamic obstruction. Systemic vascular resistance must be maintained to prevent right to left shunting across the VSD. Right ventricular emptying is usually limited by its outflow tract and not by the intrinsic pulmonary vascular resistance so nitric oxide may be of limited use. Crystalloid or non-blood colloid would usually be the fluid of choice initially in hypovolaemia since a slightly decreased pulmonary vascular resistance may help blood flow and therefore oxygen flux.

Ref: Hensley FA Jnr. The practice of cardaic anaesthesia. Chapter 13.

ANSWER 4

A. TRUE   B. TRUE   C. TRUE   D. TRUE   E. FALSE

Isolated IgA deficiency is often asymptomatic due to the effects of compensatory antibody responses, mainly secretory IgM & systemic IgG responses.

Primary hypogammaglobulinaemia is almost always associated with systemic and secretory antibody deficiencies. Deficient IgG antibody responses result in recurrent respiratory tract infections with Haemophilus, Pneumococcus or Pseudomonas and sometimes infection with some mycoplasmas and enteroviruses. It is people with cell-mediated immunity defects who get recurrent protozoal and mycobacterial infections

Ref: T.E. OH. Intensive Care Manual. Butterworths. 3rd ED, Ch 62. Immunodeficiency

ANSWER 5

A. FALSE   B. TRUE   C. FALSE   D. TRUE   E. FALSE

TUR syndrome occurs in less than 10% of TURP's. Symptoms, signs and laboratory abnormalities are caused by absorption of irrigation fluid and its subsequent metabolites, eg ammonia. Ethanol added to irrigant fluid is measured in breath or blood to give an idea of absorption. Saline disturbs the use of current from the resectoscope. It is suggested that the irrigation fluid should not be placed more than 60 cm above the patient. Glycine is suggested to act as an inhibitory neurotransmitter like GABA. Convulsions are due to profound hyponatraemia.

Ref. Miller. Anaesthesia. Transurethral resection of the prostate
Ref. Yentis, Hirsch & Smith. Anaesthesia A to Z. TURP Syndrome

ANSWER 6

A. TRUE   B. FALSE   C. TRUE   D. FALSE   E. FALSE

Scavenging systems apart from cylinders of sodalime or aldasorbers (charcoal) consist of collecting, transferring, receiving, and disposal components. The collecting system comes from a 30mm male conical fitting. These systems are of passive, semi-active and active varieties. The reservoir bag is for high expiratory flow rates, and venturi components are part of active systems. The levels of nitrous oxide should be less than 25ppm in the theatre and for halogenated agents be less than 2ppm according to US standards.

Ref: Ward. Anaesthetic equipment. Chapter 15. Atmospheric pollution.
Ref: Craft & Upton. Key topics in anaesthesia. Scavenging systems.

ANSWER 7

A. TRUE   B. FALSE   C. FALSE   D. FALSE   E. FALSE

An important recent paper has shown that the mortality is worse if pulmonary artery catheters are used in a wide group of patients, especially many of those appropriate for high dependency care. PA catheters only measure right sided pressures directly. Left atrial pressure is estimated from pulmonary artery wedge pressure. The use of too little fluid will cause an over-estimate of cardiac output by thermodilution, as may tricuspid regurgitation. In all patients pressures should be measured at end expiration.

Ref: Connors, A.F., Speroff, T., Dawson, N.V. et al (1996) The effectiveness of right heart catheterisation in the initial care of critically ill patients. JAMA. 276, 889-897.

ANSWER   8

A. FALSE   B. TRUE   C. TRUE   D. FALSE   E. TRUE

The predominant effect of dopamine on the cerebral circulation is vasodilatation with minimal $CMRO_2$ change, and at high doses there may be vasoconstrictive effects. Despite inconsistencies in available information narcotics have little effect on CBF and $CMRO_2$. When changes occur the general pattern is one of modest reductions in both CBF and $CMRO_2$. Sufentanil at low doses does not significantly affect the cerebral circulation but at doses of 10 mcg/Kg both CBF and $CMRO_2$ decrease by 25-35%. The majority of intravenous anaesthetic agents, with the exception of ketamine, produce a parallel reduction in CBF and $CMRO_2$. All the volatile agents produce variable reductions in $CMRO_2$ whilst simultaneously causing a variable increase in CBF. The benzodiazepines cause parallel reductions in both CBF and $CMRO_2$

Ref: Miller. Anesthesia. Churchill Livingstone. 4th Ed, Ch 21

ANSWER   9

A. TRUE   B. FALSE   C. TRUE   D. TRUE   E. FALSE

Severity of illness scoring systems are used to audit outcomes and adjust for case-mix differences between ICUs. They are sometimes helpful in planning an individual patients management but should not be used to decide on the withdrawal or witholding of intensive care. TISS is a measure of treatment, scoring interventions and monitoring. It assumes that severity of illness is related to treatment and monitoring intensity. It does however depend on an individual units policy on management and is probably a better indicator of nursing workload. APACHE II is the most widely used APACHE score although APACHE III is available. It uses 12 physiological variables that are weighted for the severity of their abnormality. The worst values are used. This gives an acute physiology score. To this is added a chronic health evaluation of age and premorbid illness score. The APACHE score can then be entered into an equation that includes a weighting for acute diagnosis to give a population mortality risk (not individual) for patients with this illness. SAPS II incorporates age, chronic disease, type of admission and 12 physiological measurements/investigations. It is not weighted for individual diagnosis but is easier to calculate than the APACHE II score. There are some specific trauma scoring systems. The Glasgow Coma Scale (GCS) is well known for use with head injuries. The trauma score is based on 5 parameters - respiratory rate, respiratory effort, systolic blood pressure, capillary refill time and the GCS. The revised trauma score only measures the GCS, systolic blood pressure and the respiratory rate. There are also anatomical scoring systems: the abbreviated injury scale (AIS), and the injury -severity score (ISS). Combined physiological and anatomical scoring occurs in TRISS methodology (trauma score and ISS are used).

Ref: Hillman and Bishop. Clinical Intensive Care. Cambridge University Press. Chs 3 and 14.

ANSWER   10

A. FALSE   B. TRUE   C. TRUE   D. TRUE   E. TRUE

Theophylline's elimination is enhanced by haemoperfusion, not haemodialysis, along with meprobamate, chloral hydrate, medium and short acting barbiturates. Haemodialysis is also useful in methanol poisoning. Forced alkaline diuresis is no longer recommended. As a general rule, haemodialysis is likely to enhance the excretion of substances of small molecular size that reside in high concentration in the plasma compartment (ie a small Vd).

Ref: BNF 1996; No 32: pg 20. Active elimination techniques (in Emergency treatment of poisoning. pg 18-26)

ANSWER 11

A. TRUE   B. TRUE   C. TRUE   D. TRUE   E. FALSE

Downs syndrome is present in 1/700 live births. The variety of airway problems include a small mouth, large tongue, and an increased incidence of subglottic stenosis. Atlanto-axial instability is present in 15% and is usually asymptomatic. The role of pre-operative flexion-extension radiographs is still not decided, but unless a person is symptomatic they are not universally recommended. Cardiac lesions frequently present include ASD, VSD, PDA, and tetralogy of fallot. No increased sensitivity to any group of anaesthetic agents has been demonstrated.

Ref: Miller. Anesthesia. Chapter 27. Anaesthetic implications of concurrent diseases. Chapter 42. Airway management.

ANSWER 12

A. FALSE   B. TRUE   C. FALSE   D. FALSE   E. FALSE

There is no clear evidence that one fluid is superior to the other but a greater volume of crystalloid will need to be used to obtain the same degree of intravascular resuscitation. Recent evidence from the US has shown that in patients with penetrating thoracic and abdominal trauma there appears to be an improved outcome with delayed fluid resuscitation. This has not been demonstrated with blunt trauma. Nevertheless haemorrhagic shock is the leading cause of death in multiple trauma patients, and if it occurs then mortality is doubled.

The acidosis of shock will improve with appropriate volume replacement and bicarbonate is contraindicated in acidotic states associated with tissue hypoxia as it may worsen the intracellular acidosis. Mannitol and frusemide are often given even though volume resuscitation is incomplete. There is no convincing evidence that this improves renal perfusion or can prevent or ameliorate the development of ARF. In early shock the GFR is well preserved by autoregulation, but oliguria occurs due to aldosterone and ADH secretion. As the GFR falls then the situation is compounded.

Ref: Current Anaesthesia and Critical Care 1996; Vol 7, No 3: pg 115-119. Management of major trauma: immediate care in the field. T.E. OH. Intensive Care Manual. Butterworths. 3rd Ed. Ch 58. Hypovolaemic shock

ANSWER 13

A. TRUE   B. TRUE   C. TRUE   D. TRUE   E. TRUE

Almost any drug can cause an otherwise unexplained pyrexia. Some drugs can give rise to disease of which fever may be a presenting feature e.g. antibiotic-induced colitis (clindamycin), drug induced SLE (hydralazine), drug related hepatitis (halothane) and infection consequent upon agranulocytosis caused by drugs (chloramphenicol). Hypersensitivity has been cited as the cause of many febrile reactions to drugs but frequently the evidence is not convincing.

Fever commonly follows the injection of streptokinase, this has been attributed to the release of unspecified metabolites during thrombolysis. Fever may not be due to the active agent but to other components of the product, the most common example being vaccines. Fever can follow anti-neoplastic therapy, paricularly following bleomycin and asparginase. These are derived from micro-organisms and endotoxin contamination as well as acute tumour lysis may explain the febrile occurences seen. Atropine overdose also commonly causes pyrexia, which has been attributed to the prevention of sweating, but the evidence for this is lacking. Two other examples of drug induced pyrexia are the malignant neuroleptic syndrome and malignant hyper-thermia.

Ref: Weatherall, Ledingham & Warrell. The Oxford Textbook of Medicine. Oxford Medical Publications. 3rd Ed. pg 1181-1182. Drug induced increases of body temperature.

ANSWER 14

A. FALSE   B. FALSE   C. TRUE   D. TRUE   E. TRUE

Direct measurement allows beat-by-beat assessment of arterial pressure. A continuous flush device is used that delivers 2-3ml/hr through the cannula. Damping within the measurement system should be optimal, rather than critical as the latter does not allow a fast enough response to see a normal waveform and an accurate systolic pressure. Accurate reproduction of amplitude is easy for the mean but more difficult for systolic and diastolics. Systems in clinical use, commonly have a natural frequency of 15Hz. When undamped, sine waves are reproduced accurately up to driving frequencies of only about 20% of the natural frequency (ie 3Hz). Optimal damping allows reproduction of sine waves to within to 2% of their original AMPLITUDE at driving frequencies of up to 10Hz (ie 2/3 of the natural frequency of the system). When heart rate rises or examination of the SHAPE of the waveform is critical, optimally damped systems with natural frequencies of up to 60Hz may be required.

Ref: Parbrook, G.D. and Gray, W.M. (1990) The Measurement of Blood Pressure. In: Scurr, C., Feldman, S. and Soni, N. (Eds.) Scientific Foundations of Anaesthesia; The Basis of Intensive Care, 4th edn. pp. 70-81. Oxford: Heinemann Medical Books. Nimmo & Smith. Anaesthesia. Ch27. (Blackwell).

ANSWER 15

A. FALSE   B. TRUE   C. TRUE   D. FALSE   E. TRUE

Indications for liver transplantation include end-stage liver failure secondary to inherited disease, chronic hepatitis, active toxic hepatitis, primary biliary cirrhosis and some cases of isolated liver tumour not amenable to resection. In adults, venovenous bypass is employed between the femoral and portal veins to the axillary vein, to aid venous return upon IVC cross-clamping. During the anhepatic phase hypocalcaemia occurs secondary to citrate chelation, since the citrate load in blood and blood products transfused cannot be metabolised. It is therefore standard to infuse calcium. Reperfusion of the donor liver causes transient and sometimes profound hyperkalaemia, which is usually fairly short-lived. Prolonged hypokalaemia is seen for 48 hours post-operatively as the functioning hepatocytes take up potassium. Nitrous oxide is avoided because of the risk of enlarging air emboli and to prevent bowel distension.

Ref: Yentis Hirsch and Smith. Anaesthesia A to Z. Butterworth Heinemann.

ANSWER 16

A. TRUE   B. FALSE   C. TRUE   D. TRUE   E. TRUE

Cardiac tamponade may be caused by a large pericardial effusion. Sarcoidosis is a granulomatous disorder not associated with rheumatoid arthritis. Caplans syndrome is the presence of nodular pulmonary fibrosis in patients with rheumatoid arthritis who are exposed to various industrial dusts. Ankle oedema is often seen in active rheumatoid arthritis and is caused by increased vascular permeability. Glove and stocking sensory loss is due to a polyneuropathy which causes sensory and sometimes motor loss. It is usually symmetrical and often involves the legs.

Ref: Kumar & Clark. Clinical Medicine. Balliere Tindall. Ch8

ANSWER   17

A. FALSE   B. FALSE   C. TRUE   D. FALSE   E. TRUE

First degree burns are superficial and characterised by pain and erythema, not blistering. Second degree or partial thickness burns have a red mottled appearance with swelling and blisters. Third degree or full thickness burns are dry, dark, leathery, mottled and may appear waxy. The "rule of nines" is a guide to determine the extent of the burn. The head represents ~9% BSA in adults and ~18% in infants. The larynx protects the subglottic airway from direct thermal injury but the supraglottis is susceptible to obstruction as a result of a burn. Indicators of inhalational injury include facial burns, singed eyebrows and nasal vibrissae, carbon deposits in the oropharynx, carbonaceous sputum and a history of explosion. Electrical burns can be more serious than apparent. The body may serve as a conductor of electrical energy and the heat generated injures tissue. This may result in muscle necrosis and rhabdomyolysis.

Intravenous fluid is essential in the management of 2nd and 3rd degree burns. A urine output of 1ml/kg/hr in the absence of an osmotic diuresis is the aim.

Ref. Advanced Trauma Life Support Student Manual. American College of Surgeons.

ANSWER   18

A. FALSE   B. FALSE   C. TRUE   D. TRUE   E. TRUE

In sickle cell disease, anaemia occurs from about the fourth month of life when red cells containing foetal haemoglobin (HbF) give way to adult haemoglobin (HbS). Only HbS is affected by the amino acid substitution. Cardiomegaly is a result of severe anaemia. Sickling crises are precipitated by cold, dehydration, hypoxia and infection. Both sickle cell trait and disease offer equal protection against falciparum malaria. In the West most patients survive into adulthood, but are subject to recurrent ill health and are unlikely to reach old age.

Ref: Macleod, Edwards & Bouchier. Davidsons Priciples and Practice of Medicine. 17th edition. Churchill Livingstone. Chapter: Disorders of the blood and blood-forming organs.

ANSWER   19

A. TRUE   B. TRUE   C. FALSE   D. FALSE   E. FALSE

The major changes which adversely affect gas exchange during anaesthesia are a reduced minute volume of ventilation, increased deadspace and shunt. Increased shunt in anaesthetised patients results from pulmonary collapse, decreased hypoxic pulmonary vasoconstriction and underventilation. During anaesthesia, in spontaneously breathing patients, anaesthetic agents will reduce minute ventilation, and although there is a reduced oxygen consumption $PaCO_2$ will still rise. Despite some inhaled agents being irritant, all lead ultimately to brochodilatation. However as a result of the fall in FRC, compliance is reduced.

Ref: Nunn JF. Applied Respiratory Physiology 4th ed. Butterworths. Ch 19 pp 350

ANSWER   20

A. FALSE   B. TRUE   C. TRUE   D. FALSE   E. TRUE

90% of malignancies of the oesophagus are squamous cell in origin, only 1% being adenocarcinomas. Plummer-Vinson syndrome consists of iron-deficiency anaemia and dysphagia due to a post-cricoid web in the oesophagous, which predisposes to carcinoma. Spread of oesophageal carcinoma is primarily local and lymphatic. Distant blood-borne spread is rare. Invasion into adjacent trachea can lead to tracheo-oesophageal fistula and infiltration into the recurrent laryngeal nerves can cause hoarseness.

Ref: Dunn & Rawlinson. Surgical Diagnosis and Management. Blackwell Scientific Publications.

ANSWER 21

A. FALSE   B. FALSE   C. FALSE   D. TRUE   E. TRUE

Colonic diverticula are acquired outpouchings of colonic mucosa through the bowel wall associated with increased intraluminal pressure. Almost all occur in the sigmoid and the rectum is usually unaffected. The condition is rare before middle age and in those who eat a diet high in fibre. Patients classically complain of colicky left iliac fossa pain, alteration of bowel habit or rectal bleeding.

Ref: McLatchie. Oxford Handbook of Clinical Surgery. Oxford University Press.

ANSWER 22

A. TRUE   B. TRUE   C. FALSE   D. TRUE   E. TRUE

Automaticity in the sino-atrial node is not determined by any one ion. It is determined by a mixture of Ca^{++}, K^+ and background currents. The action potential is of different form in different parts of the heart and conduction occurs at different speeds between 0.05 m/sec in the sino-atrial node and 3 m/sec in the purkinje fibres. Isoflurane in an isolated or autonomically blocked heart slows the rate of phase 4 depolarisation and slows sinus rate. This is in comparison to its effects on the intact heart.

Ref: Priebe & Skarvan. Cardiovascular Physiology. BMJ Publishing. Chapter 3. Cardiac Electrophysiology.

ANSWER 23

A. TRUE   B. FALSE   C. TRUE   D. TRUE   E. FALSE

Train of four = 4 supramaximal stimuli at 2Hz with a fixed pulse width of 0.2 ms. Force of contraction continues to slightly increase above the supramaximal threshold as a result of direct muscle stimulation. Therefore delivered current should ideally be 10-20% above the threshold. A train of four stimuli is used to detect fade on repetitive stimulation following non-depolarizing blockade. Fade is due to to non-depolarizer blockade of pre-junctional ACh receptors (which maintain ACH output with repetitive nerve stimulation). Post tetanic facilitation enables a response to occur when none was detectable following single twitches or TO4. The post tetanic count consists of a 5s 50Hz stimulus followed by a 3s pause and then single twitches at 1Hz. The number of detectable twitches is inversely related to intensity of block. Double burst stimulation = 3 x 50Hz stimuli separated by 0.75s.

ANSWER 24

A. TRUE   B. TRUE   C. FALSE   D. FALSE   E. TRUE

Rheumatoid disease affects up to 2-5% of the population. In relation to anaesthesia it has severe effects on the axial skeleton, other joints affecting the airway, on the cardiovascular and respiratory systems, on the kidney and on the immune sytem and haematological function. The cervical spine is commonly fixed in flexion with vertebral erosions and subluxation.

Temporo-mandibular joint problems commonly lead to limited mouth opening. Cricoarytenoid problems may occur in 25% of patients resulting in a narrowed glottic opening. Severe disease may affect the rest of the axial skeleton and it has been suggested that in severe disease regional blockade of the spinal cord should not be performed because of the risk of spinal fracture and cord injury. If the patient is to be asleep and has severe neck or other level disease then sensory evoked potentials may make positioning safer. Respiratory stiffness may be very significantly contributed to by chest wall stiffness from costo-chondral and other joint disease. Vasculitis is commonly present and forms the basis of much of the cardiovascular disease with cardiac failure and angina.

Ref: Katz. Anaesthesia and uncommon diseases. Connective tissue diseases.

ANSWER 25

A. FALSE **B. FALSE** **C. TRUE** **D. TRUE** **E. FALSE**

Living related donor and spousal related donor grafts have similar one year survivals, both being greater than cadaveric grafts. Size is not important but blood group and HLA antigens are. Cyclosporin toxicity oftens presents as convulsions. Patients in CRF suffer from osteoporosis and may have platelet abnormalities.

Ref: Belani KG. Kidney transplantation. Int Anes Clinics 29.pp17-39

ANSWER 26

A. TRUE **B. FALSE** **C. TRUE** **D. FALSE** **E. TRUE**

Suxamethonium does not induce an exaggerated hyperkalaemic response for the first 24-48 after a burn until proliferation of extra-junctional acetylcholine receptors has occurred, however this does not preclude the presence of hyperkalaemia from other causes. Suxamethonium should be avoided for 2-3 years after all the skin has healed after a major burn. Decreased sensitivity to non-depolarising relaxants is due to increased hepatic and renal clearance and an increased acetylcholine receptor population. Non-relaxant anaesthetic drugs act pharmacokinetically and dynamically in a normal fashion. While the upper airways can receive a direct thermal injury, lower airways are damaged by irritant compounds within smoke.

Ref: Miller Anesthesia. Chapter 14. Pharmacology of muscle relaxants and their antagonists.
Ref: Atkinson and Adams. Recent advances in anaesthesia and analgesia 15. Chapter 10. Aspects of thermal injury.

ANSWER 27

A. TRUE **B. TRUE** **C. TRUE** **D. TRUE** **E. TRUE**

Pleural effusion is common following one-lung ventilation and surgical dissection in the thorax, in patients who are often hypoalbuminaemic pre-operatively. Atrial fibrillation affects 10-20% post-operatively and some surgeons advocate prophylactic digoxin for all. Delayed gastric emptying occurs secondary to truncal vagotomy which is inevitable. Pneumothorax can occur in the contralateral lung to the side of surgical approach and so must be looked for! Patent chest drains should prevent pneumothorax on the operative side. Mediastinitis occurs following anastomotic leak and is often fatal.

Ref: Poston. Aids to Clinical Surgery. Churchill Livingstone.

ANSWER 28

A. TRUE   B. TRUE   C. TRUE   D. FALSE   E. TRUE

Infra-red absorption eg by carbon dioxide, nitrous oxide and volatile agents is used in capnography. The sample gas is drawn into a chamber through which half of a split infra-red beam is passed. The other half passes through a reference chamber containing air. The amount of infra-red light absorbed by the sample gas depends on the amount of, for example, carbon dioxide present and is determined by comparing the emergent beams from the sample and reference chambers. Delta waves in EEG are 4 Hz waves and may be normal in children and during sleep. A fuel cell consists of a lead anode and gold cathode. Oxygen diffuses to the cathode, picking up electrons when water is present to become hydroxide ions and combines with the lead to form lead oxide and give up the electrons. Thus current flows proportional to the number of oxygen molecules diffusing to the cathode. The train of four stimulations during neuromuscular blocking monitoring consists of four electrical pulses each at 2 Hz. The surface tension refers to the tangential force in the surface of a liquid and is defined as the force acting perpendicularly across a line of unit length. Hence its units are N/m.

Ref: Yentis, Hirsch, Smith. Anaesthesia A to Z. Butterworth Heinemann.

ANSWER 29

A. TRUE   B. TRUE   C. FALSE   D. FALSE   E. FALSE

Dual block occurs with larger doses of depolarising agents. If there is prolongation of the effects of depolarising relaxants by aminoglycoside antibiotics this may be helped by Ca^{++} ions. Monitoring using double burst stimulation to assess recovery from non-depolarising relaxants should occur with the two stimulations 750msecs apart.

Ref: Craft & Upton. Key topics in Anaesthesia. Neuromuscular blockade.
Ref: Yentis, Hirsch & Smith. Anaeasthesia A to Z. Neuromuscular blockade monitoring.

ANSWER 30

A. FALSE   B. TRUE   C. TRUE   D. TRUE   E. FALSE

The commonest causes of acute liver failure in developed countries are viral hepatitis (where the majority of patients have negative markers for hepatitis A and B) and paracetamol overdose. The latter more readily occurs at a given paracetamol ingestion if the patient takes hepatic microsomal enzyme inducers (antiepileptics and alcohol) and in those who are malnourished. Variables associated with a poor outcome include young or old age, unknown aetiology, encephalopthy (grade 3 or 4), acidosis, prolonged prothrombin time, elevated bilirubin and/or creatinine, and low factor V and/or alpha fetoprotein levels. AST levels do not indicate the course of the disease as they fall rapidly in severely affected livers. The treatment is mainly supportive whilst awaiting liver regeneration although orthotopic liver transplantation may be appropriate. Although up to 80% of patients develop sepsis, fever and leucocytosis are not always helpful in diagnosing it.

Ref: Herrera JL. Acute liver failure. Current Opinion in Critical Care 1996;2:134-139.

ANSWER 31

A. TRUE   B. FALSE   C. FALSE   D. FALSE   E. TRUE

Multi resistant staphylococci are now not only methicillin resistant (and therefore flucloxacillin resistant) but also gentamicin resistant. Their prevalence in Europe is increasing and they are only regularly susceptible to a glycopeptide antibiotic (vancomycin or teicoplanin). Pneumococci are increasingly resistant to penicillin. Although this is more of a problem in Spain and South Africa, it is probably inappropriate to treat a critically ill patient with penicillin. Decreased susceptibility to third generation cephalosporins and carbapenems (imipenem and meropenem) is also seen. Enterococci are the second commonest cause of nosocomial infection in the ICU. They are resistant to tetracycline, trimethoprim, chloramphenicol, penicillins, aminoglycosides and clindamycin. Vancomycin has been the antibiotic of choice but there are now vancomycin resistant enterococci (VRE) emerging. Acenetobacter spp are one of the most important Gram negative ITU pathogens. They are resistant to almost all antibiotics apart from the carbapenems. Some are still sensitive to the 4-quinolones (ciprofloxacin etc.) but this advantage is quickly lost if they are used to treat outbreaks.

Ref: Amyes SGB, Thomson CJ. Antibiotic resistance in the ICU. British Journal of Intensive Care 1995;5:263-271

ANSWER   32

A. FALSE   B. FALSE   C. TRUE   D. TRUE   E. FALSE

Epidural administration of local anaesthetics (LAs) and opioids have been used for pain relief for many years, however more recently the addition of other drugs has been considered. Clonidine has been shown to enhance the effects of both LAs and opioids in the epidural space. Side effects of LAs relate to nerve blockade, especially sympathetic blockade. Pruritis associated with epidural therapy is opioid mediated and is reversed by naloxone. Other side effects of opioids include respiratory depression, which may be delayed especially in the less lipophilic agents such as morphine. Systemic uptake of the epidural opioid is similar to intramuscular injection and placental transfer must be expected after use of the epidural route. The management of chronic pain includes the use of epidural analgesics, however there is no reduction of side effects if epidural opioids are used in comparison with other routes.

Ref: McQuay, H.J. (1994) Epidural analgesics. In: Wall, P.D. and Melzack, R. (Eds.) Textbook of Pain, 3rd edn. pp. 1025-1034. Edinburgh: Churchill Livingstone

ANSWER   33

A. FALSE   B. FALSE   C. FALSE   D. FALSE   E. FALSE

The ITU resident should never 'clear' a patient's cervical spine following blunt trauma. It can only be cleared with certainty by an appropriately qualified doctor (typically a senior orthopaedic surgeon) once he/she has checked the three view radiographs and has examined the conscious patient. If the patient is not alert then full precautions should be continued. In the unconscious patient cervical spine injury may need to be excluded by CT scan. In reality, however, many orthopaedic surgeons will 'clear' the cervical spine of an unconscious patient on the basis of radiographs alone.

Ref: Current Anaesthesia and Critical Care. 1996; Vol 7, No 3: pg 139-145 Care for trauma patients in the intensive care unit

ANSWER   34

A. TRUE   B. FALSE   C. TRUE   D. TRUE   E. TRUE

Sample errors may be due to time delay, air bubbles, mixing of blood from the catheter dead space. Air bubbles cause change in the PO_2 depending on the initial PO_2. It will tend to equilibrate with the PO_2 of the air bubble. Time delay leads to errors due to the continuing metabolism of the blood cells. This is minimised by rapid cooling, however in order to effect this the syringe should be placed in a mixture of water and ice to provide a large surface area for cooling. Although sodium heparin is generally acidic the buffering capacity of the blood ensures no change in pH. However there is a dilutional drop in PCO_2 so the bicarbonate calculated by the Henderson-Hasselbalch equation falls. Halothane mimics O_2 in polarographic electrodes so it may cause an artificially high PO_2.

Ref: Urbina, L.R. and Kruse, J.A. (1993) Blood Gas Analysis and Related Techniques. In: Carlson, R.W. and Geheb, M.A. (Eds.) Principles and Practice of Medical Intensive Care, pp. 235-250. Philadelphia: W B Saunders

ANSWER 35

A. TRUE   B. FALSE   C. FALSE   D. TRUE   E. FALSE

In normal individuals a restricted caloric intake over several days can depress the ventilatory response to hypoxia. In COPD patients impaired nutrition may result in respiratory muscle weakness and ventilatory failure, immunosuppression, anaemia and changes in pulmonary histology including a reduction in surfactant production. A high carbohydrate diet may precipitate respiratory failure in susceptible individuals and non-protein calories should be derived from fat in the majority as its RQ is 0.7 (compared with 1.0 for carbohydrates) and results in a reduced level of CO_2 production. A high protein intake has been found to increase ventilatory drive. While there may be specific indications for using specialised feeds, such as pulmocare, there is little evidence for improved outcome compared to standard feeds and they are much more expensive. The relative composition of Pulmocare and Ensure per 2000 ml is:-

	Pulmocare	Ensure
Carbohydrate (g)	210	290
Protein (g)	125	74
Fat (g)	184	74
Sodium (mmol)	114	74
Potassium (mmol)	98	80
mosm/kg water	490	450
kJ/ml	6.3	4.4

Ref: Current Anaesthesia and Critical Care 1996; Vol7, No2: pg 69-76. Enteral Nutrition. T.E. OH. Intensive Care Manual. Butterworths. Third Edition. Ch 81. Enteral Nutrition

ANSWER 36

A. FALSE   B. TRUE   C. TRUE   D. TRUE   E. FALSE

An infusion of 0.9% saline should be started immediately diagnosis is made, 1 litre should be infused over 30 minutes while preparations maybe being made for central venous cannulation.

An initial plasma hyperkalaemia will fall once tissue uptake is stimulated by insulin. Gastric dilatation may necessitate nasogastric tube insertion. Hypophosphataemia occurs, replacement is with potassium phosphate, 5 - 20 mmol / hour.

Ref: Yentis, Hirsch and Smith. Anaesthesia A to Z. Butterworth Heinemann. p137.

ANSWER   37

A. TRUE   B. FALSE   C. TRUE   D. TRUE   E. FALSE

The brachial plexus supplies the entire arm except the medial upper arm (supplied by the inter-costobrachial nerve, that can be blocked superficially just distal to the axilla).

Ref: Yentis, Hirsch, Smith. Anaesthesia A-Z Butterworths. pp56

ANSWER   38

A. TRUE   B. FALSE   C. FALSE   D. TRUE   E. TRUE

There are 7 basic SI units. These are the metre (length), kilogram (mass), second (time), ampere (current), kelvin (temperature), mole (amount of substance) and candela (luminous intensity). All others are derived. 2 supplementary units exist for the plane angle (unit = radian) and solid angle (unit = steradian). These are used in the definition of derived units but are not regarded as base units since they have no dimensions.

Ref: Sykes, Vickers, Hull. Principles of Measurement and Monitoring in Anaesthesia and Intensive Care. 3rd Edition. Blackwell Scientific Publications.

ANSWER   39

A. FALSE   B. FALSE   C. TRUE   D. FALSE   E. FALSE

Controversy still surrounds the treatment of severe head injury. Stabilisation of the cardiorespiratory system (including emergency non-neurosurgical surgery if required) and exclusion of other life threatening injuries should be undertaken immediately. Cerebral perfusion pressure should be maintained and this may include aggressive fluid administration (appropriately monitored). Hyperventilation is now generally avoided except in some situations. High intracranial pressure combined with evidence of excess cerebral perfusion (high jugular venous saturation) is treated by some centres in this way. Corticosteroids may be safe, but there is no evidence of efficacy in head trauma. Antibacterial prophylaxis is not warranted in those with a basal skull fracture and CSF leak according to The Infection in Neurosurgery Working Party of the British Society for Antimicrobial Chemotherapy.

Ref: Brock DG. Head trauma. Current Opinion in Critical Care 1996;2:105-108

ANSWER   40

A. TRUE   B. FALSE   C. TRUE   D. FALSE   E. TRUE

Muscle wasting and weakness are a common finding in patients undergoing prolonged intensive care. Causes include:

   i)   immobilisation
   ii)   malnutrition
   iii) catabolic response to illness
   iv)   acquired myopathies
   v)   critical illness neuropathy.
   vi)   medical conditions e.g Guillain Barre syndrome, CNS damage.
   vii) drugs e.g. corticosteroids, magnesium, aminoglycosides.
   viii) hypokalaemia and hypophosphataemia.

In addition to reversing any causes listed, treatment includes early adequate nutrition (perhaps supplemented with glutamine, ornithine alpha ketoglutarate, growth hormone and/or insulin-like growth factor-1 although evidence is not conclusive), physiotherapy, avoidance of neuro-muscular blockade and supportive care.

Ref: O'Leary MJ, Coakley JH. Weakness and wasting in the critically ill patient. Current Anaesthesia and Critical Care 1996;7:81-86.

ANSWER   41
A. FALSE   B. TRUE   C. FALSE   D. TRUE   E. TRUE

The majority of newborns respond appropriately to being warmed, dried, and stimulated. After this the first active step of resuscitation is to position the neonate appropriately and clear the airway. Adrenaline is required if the circulation is inadequate after oxygen ventilation and chest compressions at a dose of 10-30 mcg/kg iv or endotracheally. Meconium is present in the amniotic fluid of 10-20% of cases.

Ref: Pediatric Advanced Life Support - textbook. Chapter 9.

ANSWER   42
A. TRUE   B. TRUE   C. TRUE   D. FALSE   E. TRUE

Renal and mesenteric arterioles have a much higher input of adrenergic neurones than the cerebral and coronary vessels. Basal vascular tone and vascular resistance is also very variable between organs with renal arterioles having a very low basal tone. The arterioles of the skin are still able to dilate and constrict despite high resting tone. While inhibition of nitric oxide synthase increases vascular resistance in all organs the degree of increase is variable, demonstrating an input of local variability. The majority of the blood in the venous circulation is in its venules at microcirculatory level.

Ref: Priebe and Skarvan. Cardiovascular Physiology. Chapter 9. Microcirculation.

ANSWER   43
A. TRUE   B. FALSE   C. FALSE   D. FALSE   E. FALSE

Induction and intubation is a time of high risk in this type of surgery and invasive arterial monitoring is mandatory. Frusemide decreases renal oxygen consumption as sodium reabsorption is reduced. Normoglycaemia is the aim, hyperglycaemia may contribute to spinal cord ischaemia. Hypotension post cross-clamp release is usually multifactorial. Many centres extubate elective surgical patients at the end of the procedure.

Ref: Miller. Anaesthesia 4th ed.

ANSWER   44
A. TRUE   B. TRUE   C. FALSE   D. TRUE   E. FALSE

Cerebral perfusion pressure equals mean arterial pressure minus intracranial pressure. Cerebrovasodilators increase cerebral blood volume and can increase intracranial pressure. As a result, drugs known to increase cerebral blood flow may actually reduce it if they greatly elevate intracranial pressure. The exponential shape of the intracranial pressure : volume curve allows prediction of the likely effects on cerebral perfusion of changes in intracranial volume and pressure.

Ref : Miller. Anaesthesia 3rd ed.pp 1897

ANSWER 45

A. FALSE   B. TRUE   C. TRUE   D. FALSE   E. TRUE

Functional acute renal failure (hepatorenal syndrome) is a complication of liver failure and is characterized by intense renal vasoconstriction and sodium retention and eventually oliguric renal failure. Increased production of a number of renal vasoconstrictors including thromboxane and endothelin, and of systemic vasodilators including nitric oxide, has been demonstrated. Liver transplantation restores normal renal function and transplanted kidneys taken from patients dying from liver failure function normally.

Ref: Current Anaesthesia and Critical Care 1996; Vol 7, No 4: pg 176-181. Physiology and pathophysiology of fluids and electrolytes.

ANSWER 46

A. TRUE   B. FALSE   C. TRUE   D. FALSE   E. FALSE

ADH is secreted from the posterior pituitary, usually in response to increased plasma osmolarity. However it is secreted as part of the stress reponse to surgery and causes a fall in the total quantity of urine passed, whilst increasing the tonicity i.e. the amount of sodium excreted. Its primary site of action is in the distal tubule and collecting duct where it increases passive reabsorption of water.

Ref: Harrison, Healy and Thornton. Aids to Anaesthesia. Churchill Livingstone. pp146.

ANSWER 47

A. TRUE   B. FALSE   C. FALSE   D. TRUE   E. TRUE

TPN-induced hepatobiliary complications in children tend to be cholestatic whereas adults tend to favour steatosis and steatohepatitis (fatty changes). Biliary sludging and gall stone formation also occur. The aetiology is not clear although free amino acids may be to blame.

Elevation of transaminases (and sometimes alkaline phosphatase and bilirubin) in adults occurs later than histopathological changes, but peaks at 2 weeks and may then improve despite continued infusion.

Ref: Herrera JL. Hepatobiliary abnormalities in the critically ill. Current Opinion in Critical Care 1995;1:147-151

ANSWER 48

A. FALSE   B. FALSE   C. TRUE   D. FALSE   E. TRUE

Vitamin B12 deficiency is inevitable post-gastrectomy (lack of secreted intrinsic factor) but folate deficiency is unusual in the face of adequate nutrition. Loss of the acidic gastric environment can reduce iron and calcium absorption. Diarrhoea occurs as part of the dumping syndrome. Post-operative pancreatitis occurs and can be life-threatening.

Ref: Bailey and Love. Short practise of Surgery. Lewis and Co.

ANSWER 49

A. FALSE   B. FALSE   C. FALSE   D. TRUE   E. FALSE

MUGA involves the use of technetium-99 labelled red cells. It is used to determine peak systolic volume in relation to diastolic volume and can detect regional wall motion abnormalities. This is achieved by collecting a series of counts with a gamma camera which have been time marked against the ECG complexes, it thus requires a regular cardiac rhythm. Counts from epochs of 30-50 ms within each cardiac cycle are summated over a period of time to give an overall picture of cardiac function. Preoperative ejection fraction of <35% by MUGA has been shown to correlate with early perioperative infarction (Pasternack).

Myocardial perfusion may be assessed using the potassium analogue thallium-201. It is injected into a vein and is taken up by myocytes in proportion to the perfusion and viability of the cell. Stress can be induced by exercise or administration of dobutamine. Ischaemia may be provoked using dipyridamole or adenosine which create steal by vasodilatation of normal circulation. Reversibility of a perfusion defect demonstrates a non-infarcted area that may benefit from grafting.

Ref: Kaufman L. Anaesthesia Review 10. (Churchill Livingstone) Ch1.

ANSWER 50
A. FALSE B. TRUE C. FALSE D. FALSE E. FALSE

Barbiturates reduce intracranial pressure by reducing cerebral blood flow secondary to a fall in the cerebral metabolic rate of oxygen. A fall in the cerebral perfusion pressure (CPP) may need to be countered. Mannitol has several potential modes of action. It is an osmotic diuretic and will draw fluid from the extracellular space if the blood brain barrier is intact. However, it also reduces cerebral blood flow due to the reduction of blood viscosity and acts as a free radical scavenger. Combined with small doses of frusemide, there is a synergistic effect on ICP.

Nitrous oxide raises ICP as vasodilatation causes an increase in cerebral blood volume.

Most recent studies indicate that opioids leave cerebral blood flow unchanged or may increase it. It is thought that this is due to vasodilatation.

Ref: North B, Reilly P. Measurement and manipulation of intracranial pressure. Current Anaesthesia and Critical Care 1994;5:23-28

ANSWER 51
A. FALSE B. TRUE C. FALSE D. TRUE E. TRUE

Placental transfer of local anaesthetic agents is dependent in the first instance on maternal plasma concentration and degree of protein binding. The drug pKa and prevailing pH determine degree of ionization of free drug. Unbound unionized drug can cross into the foetal circulation. Foetal acidosis will then shift the equilibrium in favour of drug ionization trapping it within the foetal circulation. The concentration of bupivacaine measured in the umbilical vein has been shown to be only 20-35% of the maternal venous concentration because 94% within the mother is plasma protein bound. On the other hand lignocaine umbilcal vein concentrations are 70% that found in the maternal venous blood resulting in reduced neonatal neurobehavioural scores. Uterine blood flow is unaffected by extradural analgesia unless hypotension occurs.

Ref: Nimmo & Smith. Anaesthesia, Vol 1, Ch 38 (Blackwell).

ANSWER 52
A. TRUE B. TRUE C. TRUE D. FALSE E. TRUE

The majority of amino acids after deamination can be converted into acetyl-CoA from which acetoacetate can be formed. Fatty acid degradation occurs largely in the liver where acetyl-Coa is formed leading to acetoacetate production. This is transported at low levels but with efficient flux to the rest of the body. Ketosis, the presence of excessive levels of acetoacetate, beta-hydroxybutyrate or acetone in the blood can arise in starvation, diabetes mellitus or in a very largely fat based diet. Sufficient oxaloacetate is needed to receive acetyl-CoA into the citric acid cycle. Ketoacids are easily excreted by the kidney but being strong acids they are excreted combined with Na^+ from the extracellular fluid. The resultant hyponatraemia leads to an increased acidosis beyond that occasioned by the direct rise in ketoacid levels.

Ref: Guyton and Hall. Textbook of Medical Physiology. Chapter 69. Protein metabolism. Chapter 68. Lipid metabolism. Chapter 78. Insulin, glucagon and diabetes mellitus.

ANSWER 53

A. TRUE B. FALSE C. TRUE D. FALSE E. TRUE

Infra-red absorption allows measurement of many respiratory gases, but not oxygen which may actually cause interference in the measurement of carbon dioxide. Raman scattering and mass spectrometry can be used to assess all the respiratory gases. However whereas the gas can be returned unchanged after Raman scattering, mass spectrometry is destructive and the gas cannot be reused. Calorimetry measurement is used in the FEF detector for use as coarse measure of carbon dioxide. It is small, disposable and has no moving or electronic parts, so it is ideal for paramedical use in the field.

Ref: Blunt, M.C. and Urquhart, J.C. (1997) The Anaesthesia Viva: Physics, Measurement, Clinical Anaesthesia, Anatomy and Safety, London: Greenwich Medical Media.

ANSWER 54

A. TRUE B. FALSE C. TRUE D. FALSE E. TRUE

Heparin is naturally occurring and is found in mast cells. Commercial preparations are obtained from bovine or porcine lung tissue. Hypersensitivity reactions are therefore possible. Anaphylactic shock may occur, and a Type II reaction may cause severe thrombocytopaenia.

Heparin binds to antithrombin III and encourages it to inactivate thrombin. Other activated clotting factors (IXa, XIa and XIIa) and even platelets may be affected in higher doses.

Heparin lowers plasma triglceride levels. Protamine reverses the action of heparin by neutralizing the large number of anionic groups that are essential for its action.

Ref: Calvey and Williams. Principles and Practice of Pharmacology for Anaesthetists. Blackwell Scientific Publications. Ch 15.

ANSWER 55

A. FALSE B. TRUE C. FALSE D. TRUE E. TRUE

Auto-PEEP is the difference between alveolar pressure and external airway pressure at end expiration. It will occur when there is continued expiratory flow at end expiration. This possibility increases as:

i) minute volume increases– either because a larger tidal volume takes longer to empty or a higher frequency reducing the expiratory time for a set tidal volume.

ii) high expiratory resistance e.g. obstructive disease, circuit narrowing.

iii) the I:E ratio is increased as expiratory time is reduced.

Auto-PEEP can be measured by performing an expiratory hold manoeuvre and subtracting the set PEEP from the actual airway pressure at the end of this hold. This procedure is only possible in passive patients. Auto-PEEP increases peak alveolar pressure in volume controlled ventilation, reduces tidal volume in pressure controlled ventilation, interferes with pressure triggered spontaneous ventilation, increases the risk of cardiovascular instability and increases the risk of ventilator induced lung injury. Auto-PEEP can be reduced by attention to the above mentioned causative factors. Often it cannot be removed entirely without affecting the oxygenation of a critically ill patient. In these conditions, the minimum auto-PEEP with acceptable ventilation should be aimed for.

Ref: Slutsy AS (Chairman). Consensus conference on mechanical ventilation- January 28-30, 1993 at Nothbrook, Illinois, USA. Intensive Care Medicine 1994;20:64-79, 150-162

ANSWER   56

A. TRUE   B. TRUE   C. TRUE   D. FALSE   E. FALSE

All patients taking long acting sulphonylureas should be admitted to hospital several days prior to surgery and stabilised on soluble insulin. The same is true for poor diabetic control or if major surgery is planned. Ether and cyclopropane can both cause hyperglycaemia but most volatile agents in current use have little or no effect on blood glucose.

Ref: Calvey and Williams. Principles and Practice of Pharmacology for Anaesthetists. Blackwell Scientific Publications. Ch16

ANSWER   57

A. TRUE   B. TRUE   C. TRUE   D. TRUE   E. TRUE

Cholangitis can lead to bile duct narrowing and the features of obstructive jaundice. Eventually secondary biliary cirrhosis and portal hypertension result. Pyoderma gangrenosum, though rare is almost specific for ulcerative colitis or Crohns. Initially there are fluid filled intra-epidermal bullae containing a purulent fluid which burst leaving denuded areas which may colonise. Oral moniliasis requires treatment to prevent spread to the lung or oesophagus. Patients with ulcerative colitis are prone to suffer from ankylosing spondylitis. Those with both conditions belong to the HLA-B27 group, whereas those with UC do not differ from the general population.

Ref: Weatherall, Ledingham & Warrell. Oxford Textbook of Medicine. 2nd edition. Vol 1 section 12.126-12.132.

ANSWER   58

A. FALSE   B. TRUE   C. FALSE   D. FALSE   E. FALSE

Pressure controlled ventilation has become increasingly popular recently for the treatment of diseases including the acute respiratory distress syndrome (ARDS). Despite its potential advantages, there is little evidence to date that it reduces mortality or morbidity.

Advantages include:

i)   constant pressure during the inspiratory cycle which increases mean airway pressure and can lead to alveolar recruitment.

ii)   early maximal inflation of lung units that may improve gas mixing.

iii) limitation on peak airway pressure hopefully reducing the risk of ventilator induced lung injury.

iv) possibly a reduction in dysynchrony (fighting the ventilator) in those patients with a high respiratory drive due to a high inspiratory flow.

Potential disadvantages include cardiovascular instability due to venous return impairment (high mean airway pressure), loss of a guaranteed tidal volume, and possibly injury due to the high shearing forces due to the high flow at the onset of inspiration. Inspiratory flow during pressure control ventilation is of a decelerating type and is not set by the physician.

Ref: Stewart TE, Slutsky AS. Mechanical ventilation: a shifting philosophy. Current Opinion in Critical Care 1995;1:49-56

ANSWER 59
A. TRUE   B. TRUE   C. FALSE   D. TRUE   E. FALSE

The most common organisms causing meningitis are now Strep. Pneumoniae, N. Meningitidis and gram-ve bacilli. H.Influenzae type b is becoming less common due to immunization. As many as 25% of pneumococci may be resistant to penicillin, and 9% to cefotaxime. These strains can be effectively treated with a combination of rifampicin and vancomycin. Pneumococcal immunization protects against the majority of these resistant isolates. The use of dexamaethasone is controversial. It reduces long term morbidity (hearing loss) in infants and children with H. influenzae type b and may reduce mortality and morbidity in those with pneumococcal disease. However, it is unwise to use this drug if the aetiological agent is in doubt due to the risks of inappropriate antibiotic cover. If given, it should be administered 20 minutes before the antibiotics are started. The dose is 0.15mg/kg 6 hourly for 4 days. Lumbar puncture is contra-indicated in suspected cases of raised intracranial pressure. Intensive Care may be required. Tracheal intubation is undertaken for airway protection, control of intracranial pressure, ventilation if required (beware the unrousable patient), hypoxia or shock.

Ref: Roos KL, Frank M. Infectious diseases of the nervous system. Current Opinion in Critical Care 1996;2:98-104

ANSWER 60
A. TRUE   B. TRUE   C. TRUE   D. TRUE   E. TRUE

There are many medical diseases that may mimic an acute abdomen and the anaesthetist must be alive to the possibility of a primary medical diagnosis.

Ref: Hope et al. Oxford Handbook of Clinical Medicine. Oxford University Press.

ANSWER 61
A. FALSE   B. FALSE   C. TRUE   D. FALSE   E. TRUE

Adequate resuscitation of at risk patients with fluid and if necessary inotropes reduces the incidence and severity of ARF. The aim of resuscitation is to increase oxygen delivery to the kidney. The cells that are particularly susceptible are those in the ascending limbs of the loop of Henle as they are relatively poorly oxygenated at the best of times.

The major effect of dopamine on renal blood flow appears to result from an increase in cardiac output rather than a specific effect on renal blood flow. Much of the increase in urine output commonly seen with dopamine is not caused by an increased GFR but by a dopamine-mediated reduction in tubular sodium and water reabsorption. There is very little evidence that prophylactic dopamine reduces the incidence of ARF in humans, and it may be harmful by inducing cardiac arrhythmias, ischaemia, depression of thyroid function and prolactin mediated inflammatory response. Despite the perceived fear that noradrenaline may constrict renal arteries and worsen or precipitate ARF, as it does in normal individuals, it has now been shown that if noradrenaline is given to septic patients who are already on dobutamine then GFR increases and the incidence of ARF declines. Mannitol induces an osmotic diuresis if renal function is normal and is used to reduce cerebral oedema. Despite the widely held belief of its usefulness in jaundiced patients a randomised control trial looking at the effects of mannitol on postoperative renal function in patients with obstructive jaundice showed that mannitol was ineffective in preventing ARF. The loop diuretics have a theoretical advantage in the management and prevention of ARF by reducing oxygen consumption in the ascending limb of the loop of Henle by inhibiting active sodium reabsorption. If used, relatively large doses are required, e.g. 120 - 800 mg frusemide, and they do potentiate the nephrotoxicity of many other drugs. Anecdotal reports from a number of different sources suggest that the so-called Charing Cross protocol, decribed by Bullingham and Palazzo for renal rescue in the critically ill, may be effective.

Ref: British Journal of Hospital Medicine 1996; Vol 55, No 4: pg 162-166. Prevention of acute renal failure.

Ref: Current Anaesthesia and Critical Care 1996; Vol 7, No 4: pg176 - 181.Physiology and pathophysiology of fluids and electrolytes: Basic principles.

ANSWER 62
A. TRUE   B. TRUE   C. FALSE   D. FALSE   E. FALSE

The capnograph is a valuable monitor that provides more information than the adequacy of artificial ventilation. In paediatric practice with high respiratory rates the sidestream analyser may not allow clearance of CO_2 from the system during the inspiratory phase (baseline). The capnograph will fall rapidly upon the onset of ventricular fibrillation, but may show pulsation during oesophageal ventilation due to carbon dioxide from carbonated drinks or after mask ventilation. An increase in respiratory dead space may lead to a fall in the end-tidal CO_2, and this tends to lead to a significant difference in the end-tidal and arterial carbon dioxide in patients with respiratory disease.

Ref: Paulus, D.A. (1993) Noninvasive Monitoring of Oxygen and Carbon Dioxide. In: Carlson, R.W. and Geheb, M.A. (Eds.) Principles and Practice of Medical Intensive Care, pp. 203-220. Philadelphia: W B Saunders

ANSWER 63
A. TRUE   B. FALSE   C. FALSE   D. FALSE   E. TRUE

Nipple retraction or skin tethering suggests carcinoma. A breast lump may disappear after aspiration to yield clear fluid and no further treatment is necessary. If the fluid is blood stained or the lump persists urgent excision biopsy is warranted. No lump should be left without investigation. Anti-oestrogen therapy (eg Tamoxifen) is of use in the treatment of breast carcinoma.

Ref: Ellis & Calne. Lecture Notes on General Surgery. Blackwell Scientific Publications.

ANSWER 64
A. TRUE   B. TRUE   C. FALSE   D. TRUE   E. FALSE

Hypokalaemia (potassium less than 3.6 mmol/l) may lead to arrythmias, ST depression, T wave inversion and a prominent U wave on the ECG. Hyponatraemia to the extent of 114 mmol/l is abnormal. The serum sodium is frequently 5 mmol/l less than normal in hospital patients and is a result of sick cell syndrome. Bronchial carcinoma is associated with inappropriate ADH secretion which can cause severe hyponatraemia. Hypercalcaemia over 2.6 mmol/l may lead to a shortened QT interval on ECG as well as other cardiac arrythmias and hypertension. The normal plasma CSF glucose is approximately 65% of the blood glucose. A lower CSF glucose than this, as shown, is indicative of bacterial meningitis. The normal plasma albumin is 35-50 g/l. Catabolic states such as severe sepsis, trauma, fever and malignancy lead to hypoalbuminaemia.

Ref: Marshall. Clinical Chemistry. J.B. Lippincott Company.

ANSWER 65

A. TRUE   B. FALSE   C. TRUE   D. FALSE   E. TRUE

Haemoptysis may be the only symptom of the condition. Although rheumatic heart disease is the commonest cause of mitral stenosis it may also be congenital, secondary to infective endocarditis or to SLE. In untreated severe mitral stenosis, sodium retention can occur which leads to pleural effusions, peripheral oedema, ascites or pulmonary oedema. All valvular heart disease requires prophylactic antibiotics for dental treatment. Atrial fibrillation is a feature of mitral stenosis and may lead to systemic or pulmonary emboli. A mitral thrombus may also form and so anticoagulation is recommended.

Ref: Weatherall, Ledingham & Warrell. Oxford Textbook of Medicine. 2nd edition. vol 2. Section 13.283-13.286.

ANSWER 66

A. TRUE   B. TRUE   C. TRUE   D. FALSE   E. TRUE

Hypopituitarism reduces levels of growth hormone and ACTH which cause hypoglycaemia. Failure to catabolise insulin in cirrhosis leads to hypoglycaemia. Reactive hypoglycaemia can occur post partial gastrectomy. It is thought to be caused by an excessive insulin response to a glucose load. It occurs typically some 3 hours after a meal. It is not usually enough to impair consciousness and may be treated by reducing the carbohydrate content of the diet. Catecholamine excess will cause hyperglycaemia. An insulinoma is a pancreatic islet cell tumour which can cause hypoglycaemia, confusion, loss of consciousness, seizures, diplopia, sweating and weakness. 95% are benign.

Ref: Beck, Francis & Souhami. Tutorials in Differential Diagnosis. 2nd edition. Churchill Livingstone. p132. Kumar & Clark. Clinical Medicine. Balliere Tindall. Chapter 17.

ANSWER 67

A. TRUE   B. FALSE   C. FALSE   D. FALSE   E. FALSE

The clinical criteria for the diagnosis of brain-stem death include apnoeic coma despite adequate arterial PCO_2, but do not require an isoelectric EEG. Donor spinal reflexes often persist despite brain stem death. Malignancy generally precludes organ donation unless it is limited to primary CNS malignancy. Age > 40 years precludes cardiac donation.

Ref: Yentis Hirsch and Smith. Anaesthesia A to Z. Butterworth Heinemann.

ANSWER 68

A. TRUE   **B. TRUE**   **C. FALSE**   **D. TRUE**   **E. TRUE**

For a drug interaction to occur, prior or concomitant administration of a drug modifies the effect of another in addition to summative effects. SSRI's are indirectly acting sympathomimetic amines, and hypertensive crises are possible if administered with monoamine oxidase inhibitors. Tricyclic antidepressants lower the convulsive threshold and therefore antagonise carbamazepine and phenytoin. Propofol and bolus fentanyl do not interact apart from summative effects. In contrast, propofol and alfentanil by continuous infusion result in higher than expected alfentanil levels. Lignocaine, as a base, binds to alpha-1 acid glycoprotein in the plasma. Other basic drugs can therefore displace it. Verapamil has membrane stabilising properties and can potentiate the sedative effects of benzodiazepines.

Ref: Hindle AT, Columb MO, Shah MV. Drug interactions and anaesthesia. Current Anaesthesia and Critical Care 1995;6:103-112

ANSWER 69

A. TRUE   **B. TRUE**   **C. FALSE**   **D. FALSE**   **E. FALSE**

Hepatic encephalopathy can be precipitated in those with hepatocellular failure by a number of different mechanisms including infection, gastro-intestinal haemorrhage and sedative drugs. By causing derangement of electrolytes and/or dehydration, diuretics can also promote encephalopathy. Lactulose, by reducing the length of time that protein remains in the bowel lumen, should be prescribed to keep the stool loose. In chronic hepatocellular failure, some patients are not protein intolerant, and therefore should be advised to have a high protein intake. The normocytic, normochromic anaemia is not usually due to haematinic deficiency. Occult blood loss may lead to iron deficiency. Although commonly recommended, vitamin K therapy often fails to reverse the failure of clotting factor synthesis by the liver.

Ref: Oxford Textbook of Medicine (Third Edition) Oxford University Press. Ch

ANSWER 70

A. TRUE   **B. TRUE**   **C. TRUE**   **D. FALSE**   **E. FALSE**

80% of children with pyloric stenosis are male. The metabolic alkalosis results from loss of hydrochloric acid from the stomach giving a hypochloraemic alkalosis. Dehydration and resultant hypovolaemia lead to raised aldosterone secretion which together with the alkalosis causes hypokalaemia. Aldosterone is responsible for an exchange of potassium and hydrogen ions for sodium in the urine. This results in a paradoxical acid urine.

Ref: Yentis, Hirsch & Smith. Anaesthesia A to Z. Butterworth Heinemann. p378

ANSWER 71

A. FALSE   **B. FALSE**   **C. TRUE**   **D. FALSE**   **E. FALSE**

Treatment of cancer pain is a multifactorial problem. When pain is sensitive to conventional analgesics, then the World Health Organisation recommends treating in a stepwise order, starting with a non-opioid, usually aspirin. If this fails to control the pain, a weak opioid such as codeine is added. If pain is still poorly controlled, the weak opioid is replaced by a strong opioid e.g. morphine. At all stages, adjuvant analgesics e.g. antidepressants or anticonvulsants, should be used if appropriate and effective. Analgesics should be given by mouth whenever possible. The oral dose of morphine is 2-3 times that of the injectable dose, as is the rectal dose. They should be given regularly at intervals to prevent breakthrough pain. Corticosteroids can be used for pain due to nerve compression or when a large tumour and surrounding inflammation is causing pain due to pressure. Following phenol neuroablative block, inadvertant motor block should recover in time. Alcohol, however, causes permanent motor impairment in the majority of cases.

Ref: Nimmo, Rowbotham and Smith. Anaesthesia (Second Edition) Blackwell Scientific Publications. p.1216-29

ANSWER 72

A. FALSE   B. FALSE   C. TRUE   D. TRUE   E. FALSE

Patients with ESRF often present a considerable anaesthetic problem. They are anaemic, hypertensive, coagulopathic and acidotic. They often have silent ischaemic heart disease and are treated with steroids and immunosuppressants.

Ref: Zauder. Anaesthesia for patients who have terminal renal disease. ASA refresher course 4:163—173, 1990.

ANSWER 73

A. FALSE   B. FALSE   C. FALSE   D. TRUE   E. FALSE

Randomisation means that the choice of treatment arm or group is selected without bias, It does not require any test and can be achieved in several ways.

Ref: Yentis, Hirsch and Smith. Anaesthesia. Butterworths.pp418

ANSWER 74

A. TRUE   B. TRUE   C. FALSE   D. TRUE   E. TRUE

The abducent nerve (VI) supplies the lateral rectus of the eye. It emerges through the medial side of the superior orbital fissure. The superior oblique is supplied by the trochlear nerve (IV) whereas the other ocular muscles are supplied by the oculomotor nerve (III). The lingual nerve is a sensory branch of the mandibular division of the trigeminal nerve (V). It supplies the floor of the mouth, gums and along with the chorda tympani supplies the anterior two thirds of the tongue. The ulnar nerve supplies the skin of the medial one and a half digits, the median nerve supplies the lateral three and a half digits over the palmar aspect.

The pudendal nerve from the sacral plexus (S2,3,4) supplies the skin and glans of the penis via the two dorsal nerves of the penis. The auriculo temporal nerve is a branch of the mandibular division of the trigeminal nerve (V).It supplies the tragus, the temporo mandibular joint, external auditory meatus and the tympanic membrane.

Ref. Snell. Clinical Anatomy For Medical Students. Little Brown. Boston.

ANSWER 75

A. FALSE   B. FALSE   C. FALSE   D. FALSE   E. FALSE

The anterior spinal artery is formed by the union of two branches of the vertebral artery. It supplies the anterior two-thirds of the cord. The two posterior spinal arteries arise from the posterior cerebellar arteries and supply the posterior third. Branches of the vertebral, cervical, intercostal and lumbar arteries enter the vertebral canal through the intervertebral foramina.

These spinal branches divide into anterior and posterior radicular arteries that travel along the nerve roots to reach the cord where they anastamose with the anterior and posterior spinal arteries. One of these radicular arteries is larger than the rest and represents the major supply to the lower two-thirds of the cord. It is known as the artery of Adamkiewicz and is located in the lower thoracic or upper lumbar region. It is more common on the left.

Ref. Barash, Cullen and Stoelting. Clinical Anaesthesia. 2nd edition. J.B. Lippincott Company.

ANSWER 76
A. FALSE   B. FALSE   C. TRUE   D. TRUE   E. FALSE

There are strict guidelines issued by the joint colleges regarding brain stem testing. The cause of coma must be known. There must be no evidence of metabolic or pharmacological causes for the coma. Two senior independent physicians must conduct the tests. All brainstem functions must be absent and the apnoea test positive. During the cold caloric test the eyes must not move, if this reflex is intact remember "cold away and warm towards". There is no requirement for EEG evidence.

Ref: Posner and Plum. Differential diagnosis of coma.

ANSWER 77
A. FALSE   B. TRUE   C. FALSE   D. TRUE   E. FALSE

For surgery to the foot, the tibial nerve, sural nerve, deep and superficial peroneal nerves and the saphenous nerve need to be blocked. The tibial nerve supplies the medial and lateral plantar nerves. All except the saphenous nerve (femoral) are derived from the sciatic nerve.

Ref: Yentis, Hirsch,and Smith. Anaesthesia A-Z. Butterworths. pp23

ANSWER 78
A. TRUE   B. FALSE   C. TRUE   D. TRUE   E. TRUE

AF is sometimes the only feature of thyrotoxicosis (apathetic hyperthyroidism). Anticoagulation is advised in those with chronic AF, and in paroxysmal AF, if caused by mitral valve or alcoholic heart disease because of the risk of atrial thrombosis and embolism. Both acute and chronic alcoholism can lead to AF. 'f' waves on the ECG are fine oscillations of the baseline seen in AF. No clear P waves are seen. Oral flecainide maybe used to prevent recurrent paroxysms of AF.

Ref: Kumar & Clark. Clinical Medicine. Balliere Tindall. Ch 11

ANSWER 79
A. FALSE   B. FALSE   C. TRUE   D. TRUE   E. FALSE

The right common carotid arises from the brachiocephalic artery whereas the left common carotid emerges from the aortic arch. They ascend in the carotid sheath in the neck and divide into internal and external carotids at the level of C4. The carotid sinus is a dilatation in the internal carotid just above the bifurcation. The internal carotid passes through the carotid canal at the base of the skull with the internal jugular vein. It then divides into the anterior and middle cerebral arteries. The vertebral artery is a branch of the subclavian artery.

Ref: Yentis, Hirsch and Smith. Anaesthesia A to Z. Butterworth Heinemann.

ANSWER 80

A. TRUE   B. FALSE   C. FALSE   D. FALSE   E. TRUE

The size 1 mask is appropriate for infants up to 6.5kg and should be inflated with up to 4ml; the size 2 mask for 6.5-20kg with an inflation volume up to 10ml; the size 2.5 for 20-30kg with an inflation volume up to 14ml. For cleaning, the cuff should be fully deflated immediately prior to autoclaving.

Ref: Intavent product information sheet.

ANSWER 81

A. FALSE   B. FALSE   C. FALSE   D. TRUE   E. TRUE

The distal tubule is for fine tunning and Na$^+$ can be exchanged for H$^+$. The countercurrent multiplier is to make the medulla hypertonic so increasing water reabsorption from the collecting duct.

Ref : Scurr, Feldman, Soni. Scientific Foundatiions 4th ed. Heinemann. pp 448

ANSWER 82

A. TRUE   B. FALSE   C. TRUE   D. FALSE   E. TRUE

Pre-eclampsia is a multisystem disorder of unknown aetiology and unique to pregnant women after 20 weeks gestation. The common pathological feature in the placenta, kidneys and brain is vascular endothelial damage and dysfunction. Normal pregnant women lose sensitivity to angiotensin II, whilst pre-eclamptic women develop increased sensitivity to this hormone. Thrombocytopenia occurs in one-third of pre-eclamptic women and maternal vascular prostacyclin is reduced and platelet production of thromboxane is increased. In patients with severe pre-eclampsia the cardiac index is low or normal, systemic vascular resistance is normal or very high and PCWP is either low or normal. The recent CLASP study showed that the use of aspirin did not significantly affect the incidence of proteinuria, eclampsia or IUGR. Whilst aspirin use was associated with a 12% reduction in the incidence of pre-eclampsia, this was not significant. Methyldopa is the only antihypertensive drug with documented long-term safety for the newborn, ACE inhibitors are associated with toxic effects in the fetus and are therefore contraindicated. Nifedipine is an effective first or second line treatment however there is limited data on its effects on the fetus. The side effects of hydralazine include headache, tremor and vomiting all of which are also symptoms of impending eclampsia. Magnesium sulphate is the preferred treatment of impending or established eclampsia and has a significantly lower risk of recurrent convulsions than either diazepam or phenytoin and a lower mortality rate. It is thought to reverse cerebral vasoconstriction by blocking calcium influx through the NMDA subtype of glutamate channel. Plasma concentrations exceeding 4 mmol/litre cause toxicity which can be treated with i.v. calcium gluconate 1gm.

Ref: British Journal of Anaesthesia. 1996; 76: 133-148. Recent developments in the pathophysiology and management of pre-eclampsia

ANSWER 83

A. FALSE   B. TRUE   C. TRUE   D. TRUE   E. TRUE

The JVP wave consists of 3 peaks (a, c, v) and 2 troughs (x and y descents). The order of occurence is a, c, x, v, y. The a wave is produced by atrial contraction. The x descent occurs when the atrial contraction finishes. The c wave is caused by transmission of rapidly rising right ventricular pressure before the tricuspid valve closes. The v wave is due to venous return filling the right atrium during ventricular systole. The y descent follows the v wave when the tricupid valve opens. Cannon waves are large a waves.

Ref: Kumar & Clark. Clinical Medicine. Balliere Tindall. Chapter 11

ANSWER 84

A. FALSE   B. FALSE   C. TRUE   D. FALSE   E. TRUE

Indocyanine green (Cardio-green or Fox-green) is the dye most commonly used in the dye dilution method of measuring cardiac output. This method is prone to recirculation error as dye recirculates before the original has been cleared. In the thermal indicator method this does not occur. There are respiratory fluctuations in temperature in the pulmonary artery hence injection during inspiration may give different results than during expiration. Doppler ultrasonography is useful in providing beat to beat measurements of cardiac output but is less accurate than thermodilution methods as it requires measurement of the diameter of the aorta (to calculate cross sectional area) and this varies along its length.

Ref: Sykes, Vickers, Hull. 3rd Edition. Priciples of Measurement and Monitoring in Anaesthesia and Intensive Care. Blackwell Scientific Publications.

ANSWER 85

A. FALSE   B. FALSE   C. FALSE   D. FALSE   E. TRUE

The diaphragm consists of a central tendinous trefoil and a muscular periphery. It is attached partly by the crura to the left and right. The right is larger and extends from the sides of the first to third lumbar vertebrae whereas the left extends from the first to the second. Various openings in the diaphragm exist. At the level of T12 the opening transmits the descending aorta , the azygos vein and the thoracic duct. At T10 is the oesophageal opening which also transmits the right gastric artery and the trunks of the right and left vagi. The caval opening also transmits the right phrenic nerve at T8. The phrenic nerve (C3,4,5) is the sensory and motor supply to the diaphragm with the major supply derived from C4.

Ref. Snell. Clinical Anatomy For Medical Students. Little Brown. Boston.

ANSWER 86

A. TRUE   B. TRUE   C. FALSE   D. TRUE   E. TRUE

The pulmonary artery occlusion pressure (PAOP, 'wedge', PAWP, PCWP) reflects the left ventricular end diastolic pressure (LVEDP) in most circumstances. Mitral stenosis and positive pressure ventilation raise the PAOP (the degree of alteration by the latter is dependent on pulmonary compliance). If the tip of the pulmonary artery catheter is too far advanced and lies above the left atrium, then alveolar pressure will affect the measured pressure, which will therefore be accentuated by PEEP or positive pressure ventilation (especially in hypovolaemia when the capillaries are likely to collapse). LVEDP reflects LVEDV but the latter is also determined by ventricular compliance.

Ref: Soni. Anaesthesia and Intensive Care; Practical Procedures. Heinemann Professional Publishing. Ch 1.

ANSWER 87

A. FALSE   B. FALSE   C. FALSE   D. TRUE   E. TRUE

Congenital hypertrophic pyloric stenosis leads to pyloric obstruction and subsequent projectile vomiting and dehydration. 2 children in 1000 are affected. 80% are males and 50% are first-born. It usually presents 3-6 weeks after birth and 80% have a palpable tumour with visible peristalsis. The infant is usually ravenously hungry, feeding voraciously only to vomit immediately. Adequate rehydration and correction of the hypochloraemic hypokalaemic alkalosis is vital before surgery, which is never an emergency.

Ref: Yentis Hirsch and Smith. Anaesthesia A to Z. Butterworth Heinemann.

ANSWER 88

A. TRUE   B. TRUE   C. FALSE   D. FALSE   E. TRUE

The anaemia of chronic diseases (rheumatoid arthritis, SLE, neoplasia) is normocytic and normochromic. Both the serum iron and the total iron binding capacity (TIBC) are low in contrast to the raised TIBC in iron deficiency anaemia. Iron stores are normal and hence the anaemia does not respond to iron but to the treatment of the underlying condition. Strict vegans lack vitamin B12 found in meat, fish, eggs and milk, this causes a megaloblastic anaemia. Vitamin B12 stores in the body are large compared to daily losses so it takes a long time (about 5 years) for a deficiency to develop. Alcoholism leads to a megaloblastic anaemia secondary to folate deficiency which unlike B12 deficiency develops quickly as stores are used up in about 4 months.

Ref: Kumar & Clark. Clinical Medicine. Balliere Tindall. Chapter 6

ANSWER 89

A. TRUE   B. FALSE   C. FALSE   D. TRUE   E. TRUE

Bioavailability is affected by degree of absorption and first pass metabolism and is important when switching modes of drug administration perioperatively.

Disopyramide	=	85%
Propranolol	=	10-30%
Verapamil	=	20%
Digoxin	=	55-80%
Amiodarone	=	60-80%

Ref: Oh t. Intensive Care Manual (Butterworths) Ch4.

ANSWER 90

A. FALSE   B. FALSE   C. FALSE   D. TRUE   E. TRUE

Erythrocytes are made in the bone marrow in adults. Erythropoietin is largely produced by the kidneys and hypoxia is a major stimulus for its production. Vitamin B12 is required for normal erythrocyte production.

Ref: Harrison, Healy and Thornton. Aids to Anaesthesia. Churchill Livingstone. pp194

NOTES

NOTES

QBase Anaesthesia
on CD-ROM

SYSTEM REQUIREMENTS

An IBM compatible PC with a minimum 80386 processor and 4Mb of RAM
VGA Monitor set up to display at least 256 colours
CD-ROM drive
Windows 3.1 or higher with Microsoft compatible mouse

The display setting of your computer must be set to display "SMALL FONTS". See Windows manuals for further instructions on how to do this.

INSTALLATION INSTRUCTIONS

The program will install the appropriate files onto your hard drive. It requires the QBase CD-ROM to be installed in the D:\drive.

In order to run QBase the CD-ROM must be in the drive.

Print Readme.txt and Helpfile.txt on the CD-ROM for fuller instructions and user manual

WINDOWS 95

1. Insert the QBase CD-ROM into the drive **D:**
2. From the **Start Menu,** select the **RUN option**
3. Type **D:\setup.exe and press enter or return**
4. **Follow the Full Installation** option and accept the default directory for installation of QBase.

   The installation program creates a folder called **QBase** containing the program icon and another called **Exams** into which you can save previous exam attempts.

5. To run QBase double click the **QBase** icon in the QBase folder. From Windows Explorer double click the **QBase.exe** file in the QBase folder.

WINDOWS 3.1/WINDOWS FOR WORKGROUPS 3.11

1. Insert the QBase CD-ROM into the drive **D:**
2. From the **File Menu,** select the **RUN option**
3. Type **D:\setup.exe and press enter or return**
4. Follow the instructions given by the installation program. Select the **Full Installation** option and accept the default directory for installation of QBase

   The installation program creates a program window and directory called **QBase** containing the program icon. It also creates a directory called **Exams** into which you can save previous attempts.

5. To run QBase double click on the **QBase** icon in the QBase program. From File Manager double click the **QBase.exe** file in the QBase directory